Acute Pain Management
A practical guide

Commissioning Editors: Natasha Andjelkovic, Michael Parkinson

Project Development Manager: Lulu Stader

Project Manager: Anne Dickie

Design Direction: Stewart Larking

Third Edition

Acute Pain Management
A practical guide

By
Pamela E Macintyre
BMedSc, MBBS, MHA, FANZCA, FFMANZCA

Director, Acute Pain Service
Department of Anaesthesia, Hyperbaric Medicine and Pain Medicine
Royal Adelaide Hospital
and University of Adelaide
Adelaide, Australia

Stephan A Schug
MD, FANZCA, FFPMANZCA

Professor and Chair of Anaesthesiology, Pharmacology
and Anaesthesiology Unit
School of Medicine and Pharmacology, University of Western Australia
Director of Pain Medicine, Royal Perth Hospital
Perth, Australia

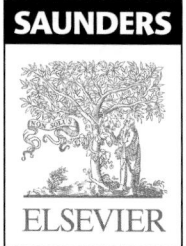

SAUNDERS

ELSEVIER

Edinburgh   London   New York   Oxford   Philadelphia   St Louis   Sydney   Toronto 2007

SAUNDERS
ELSEVIER

An Imprint of Elsevier Limited

© Elsevier Limited 2007. All rights reserved.

First edition 1996
Second edition 2001
Third edition 2007
 Reprinted 2008

ISBN 978 0 7020 2770 3

British Library Cataloguing in Publication Data
A catalogue record for this book is available from the British Library

Library of Congress Cataloging in Publication Data
A catalog record for this book is available from the Library of Congress

Notice
Knowledge and best practice in this field are constantly changing. As new research and experience broaden our knowledge, changes in practice, treatment and drug therapy may become necessary or appropriate. Readers are advised to check the most current information provided (i) on procedures featured or (ii) by the manufacturer of each product to be administered, to verify the recommended dose or formula, the method and duration of administration, and contraindications. It is the responsibility of the practitioner, relying on their own experience and knowledge of the patient, to make diagnoses, to determine dosages and the best treatment for each individual patient, and to take all appropriate safety precautions. To the fullest extent of the law, neither the Publisher nor the Authors assume any liability for any injury and/or damage to persons or property arising out or related to any use of the material contained in this book.

The Publisher

ELSEVIER your source for books, journals and multimedia in the health sciences
www.elsevierhealth.com

Working together to grow libraries in developing countries
www.elsevier.com | www.bookaid.org | www.sabre.org

ELSEVIER   BOOK AID International   Sabre Foundation

The Publisher's policy is to use **paper manufactured from sustainable forests**

Printed in China

Foreword

The first and second editions of this book struck a very receptive chord with clinicians because of the blend of rigorous evaluation of the literature and the obvious credibility of the recommendations for clinical management. This did not surprise me at all, given that the first author leads a large and successful acute pain management programme and has been a leader in research and education in this field since its inception. In the late 1990s, when I was assembling the Foundation Board for the Faculty of Pain Medicine in Australia, I selected Pam Macintyre as a Board Member because of her obvious leadership in the acute pain field and her interest in the overlap between acute and persistent pain. Also during the years 1995–1999, when I was engaged in editing Australia's first evidence-based clinical practice guideline on acute pain management, I chose Dr Macintyre to be one of the major contributors to this document.[1]

During my term as its President, the Australian and New Zealand College of Anaesthetists (ANZCA) decided to revise the 1999 document mentioned above, in collaboration with the NHMRC. Dr Macintyre was my clear choice to chair the working party that led to the revised document. She did an outstanding job in producing a summary of the scientific evidence that underpins the management of acute pain, which is currently the best source of this information worldwide.[2] Other specialist medical colleges in Australia endorsed this document, as did the International Association for the Study of Pain (IASP), and the Royal College of Anaesthetists in the United Kingdom was represented on the working party leading to the production of the guideline.

Given this background, it is not surprising that the third edition of Dr Macintyre's book is based strongly on an assessment of the scientific evidence that underpins acute pain management, but retains the very practical approach of the first and second editions. For this edition she is joined by Professor Stephen Schug as co-author. Professor Schug is Editor-in-Chief of the journal *Acute Pain,* was a key member of the working party referred to above, and directs an excellent pain service for acute, chronic and cancer pain in Perth, Western Australia. Professor Schug's strong research track record in this field nicely complements Dr Macintyre's range of expertise.

The 14 chapters that make up this book provide a comprehensive cover of all of the areas of importance in the management of acute pain. There is a new and comprehensive assessment of the patient with acute pain, which emphasizes both initial and ongoing assessment. There is also emphasis on the importance of adequately assessing the adverse effects of pain and pain treatment. In Chapter 6 on non-opioid and adjuvant analgesic agents, the increasing number of available agents receive appropriate attention.

Over the past 5 years much attention has been given in the basic and clinical pain literature to the important areas of acute neuropathic pain and the transition from acute to persistent pain. Thus the clinician is provided with a precise summary of the pathophysiology of neuropathic pain and its clinical features, as well as the various acute neuropathic pain syndromes. Current treatments for neuropathic pain are described, with a focus on the acute presentation. The reader is also given an up-to-date insight into current knowledge of the factors that predispose to progression from acute pain to persistent pain, and what can be done to prevent this undesirable outcome.

The final chapter, appropriately, deals with complex patients who require particular attention to assessment and treatment: the elderly; opioid-tolerant patients; patients with a substance abuse disorder; patients with obstructive sleep apnea; pregnant or lactating patients; and patients with renal or hepatic impairment.

At the end of the text there is a section providing self-assessment questions for the reader, and I applaud the inclusion of this material.

I congratulate Dr Macintyre and Professor Schug on providing the appropriate balance between the scientific basis of acute pain management and a concise practical summary of current options for clinical management. Acute pain management remains suboptimal; however, there have been advances over the last 5–10 years which can be attributed to the publication of professional guidelines and the availability of texts such as this.

Professor Michael J Cousins AM, MD, DSc, FANZCA, FRCA, FFPMANZCA, FAChPM(RACP)
Professor and Director
Pain Management Research Institute
University of Sydney at Royal North Shore Hospital
St Leonards
Australia 2065

References

[1]NHMRC. 1999 Acute pain management: scientific evidence. *(http://www.fpm.anzca.edu.au)*
[2]NHMRC. 2005 Acute pain management: scientific evidence. *(http://www.fpm.anzca.edu.au)*

Preface

The first edition of this book aimed to provide nurses, medical students and doctors in training (interns, house officers, residents and registrars) with simple and practical information and guidelines that would help them manage their patients' pain more effectively. It was intended to give them a better understanding of the conventional methods of analgesia as well as the newer techniques that were increasingly being used for the management of acute pain, such as patient-controlled and epidural analgesia.

The second edition updated the information in the book and added chapters to assist in the management of three groups of patients in whom acute pain management can be a little more challenging – opioid-tolerant patients, patients with acute neuropathic pain, and elderly patients.

Since the second edition, recognition of the need to improve the management of acute pain, as well as chronic and cancer pain, has continued to increase. Key international bodies such as the World Health Organization and the International Association for the Study of Pain (IASP) have highlighted that appropriate pain relief, including relief of acute pain, 'should be a Human Right'.

There have also been changes in the complexity of acute pain therapies and in the type of patient seen with acute pain. Comprehensive acute pain management does not just mean care of patients with pain from mainly postoperative, obstetric and trauma-related causes, but includes the management of patients with acute-on-chronic pain, acute cancer pain or acute pain from a multitude of medical conditions.

Knowledge relating to the treatment of acute pain has continued to grow rapidly and the quality of the evidence available has improved significantly. However, this progress has not led to the same degree of progress in patient care. Publications continue to show that the management of acute pain is often still less than optimal in both surgical and medical patients. While significant advances have been made in the understanding, assessment, and management of acute pain, this has not generally been translated into improvements in clinical practice.

The third edition of this book incorporates information on some of the many changes occurring in clinical practice. Some chapters have been extensively updated while others have been added to reflect the increasing complexity of acute pain medicine. A separate chapter on assessment and monitoring highlights the importance of regular patient assessment and the need to individualize treatment for each patient, and more information has been added to the chapters on the different drugs and techniques used in acute pain management. Chapters on postsurgical pain syndromes and acute neuropathic pain, and analgesia in specific nonsurgical states as well as for some of the more complex patient groups, have also been included.

Added to each chapter are key points that highlight the level of evidence available for that topic. The evidence has been annotated according to the system recommended by the National Health and Medical Research Council (NHMRC) of Australia. This system was also used in the production of *Acute Pain Management: Scientific Evidence* (2nd edition) by the Australian and New Zealand College of Anaesthetists (ANZCA) and the Faculty of Pain Medicine (FPM), which was endorsed by the NHMRC and the IASP.

I   Evidence obtained from a systematic review of all relevant randomized controlled trials

II   Evidence obtained from at least one properly designed randomized controlled trial

III-1 evidence obtained from well-designed pseudo-randomized controlled trials (alternate allocation or some other method)

III-2 Evidence obtained from comparative studies with concurrent controls and allocation not randomized (cohort studies), case-controlled studies or interrupted time series with a control group

III-3 Evidence obtained from comparative studies with historical control, two or more single-arm studies, or interrupted time series without a parallel control group

IV   Evidence obtained from case series, either post-test or pre-test and post-test

NHMRC (*1999*) *A guide to the development, implementation and dissemination of clinical practical guidelines*. Copyright Commonwealth of Australia reproduced by permission

---

Clinical practice points were added to the ANZCA document and related to information that was considered by the working party to be recommended best practice based on clinical experience, but for which there was no good evidence.

Both authors were members for the ANZCA/FPM working party responsible for the production of that document and we are grateful to ANZCA for permission to reproduce selected key messages in this book.

The third edition remains a practical book on adult non-obstetric acute pain management only and detailed information about the anatomy, neurochemistry and pathophysiology of acute pain has been omitted. It is not possible for a book of this size to contain comprehensive information on every drug or technique used for the management of acute pain. Suggested drugs, doses and treatment regimens are guidelines only and may have to be adapted according to different patients and clinical situations. INN drug names have been used throughout the book.

We are grateful to our anesthesiology and nursing colleagues for their comments and suggestions following the previous two editions of this book and would welcome any feedback on this third edition.

Pamela E Macintyre
Stephan A Schug
2006

Australian and New Zealand College of Anaesthetists, Faculty of Pain Medicine. (2005) Acute pain management: scientific evidence (2nd edition). Melbourne: Australian and New Zealand College of Anaesthetists,
Also available at *http://www.anzca.edu.au/publications/acutepain.htm*, and *http://www7. health.gov.au/nhmrc/publications/synopses/cp104syn.htm*
International Association for the Study of Pain, European Federation of IASP Chapters. (2004) Fact sheet: Unrelieved pain is a major global healthcare problem. Available at *http://www.painreliefhumanright.com/pdf/04a_global_day_fact_sheet.pdf*
National Health and Medical Research Council. (1999) A guide to the development, implementation and dissemination of clinical practice guidelines. *http://www7.health.gov.au/nhmrc/publications/_files/cp30.pdf*

Contents

Introduction

Over the last few years significant advances have been made in the assessment and management of acute pain. There have also been increases in the complexity and effectiveness of acute pain treatments, as well as in the quantity and quality of literature relating to the management of acute pain. However, these advances have not necessarily led to improved patient care.

Effectiveness of acute pain management

Since the 1960s, studies of adult hospital patients have consistently highlighted inadequacies in the treatment of acute pain. Despite the advances that have occurred in the intervening years, the management of acute pain remains suboptimal for many surgical and medical patients. It is thought that more than 50% of patients may still have severe pain after surgery (both in hospital and after discharge), and that more than 30% of medical patients with pain will report their pain as being severe.

Improvements in acute pain management over the last 10–20 years have been due largely to the introduction of new techniques for the delivery of analgesic

1

drugs (e.g. patient-controlled and epidural analgesia), the use of newer drugs and/or the combination of older ones as part of multimodal analgesia, and the establishment of acute pain services.

Pain relief for patients prescribed one of the more traditional analgesic techniques (e.g. intermittent intramuscular opioid analgesia) commonly remains inadequate. However, with adequate staff training, involvement of the patient, and the use of more flexible dosing regimens, even simple injections of intramuscular (IM) or subcutaneous (SC) morphine can be effective.

These factors are also important when newer methods of pain relief are used. For example, patient-controlled analgesia (PCA) can provide excellent and safe pain relief if conditions exist that facilitate its effective use. However, if a patient is just given a PCA machine, with inadequately trained nursing and medical staff and without an adequate explanation of the technique, results may be at best disappointing and at worst unsafe. Similarly, the practice of epidural analgesia without adequate and appropriate staff education, regular anesthesiology review and 24-hour backup, may also lead to problems ranging from inadequate pain relief to delayed recognition of complications such as an epidural hematoma or abscess, and therefore an increased risk to the patient of permanent neurological damage.

Improvements in acute pain management must aim at better analgesia for all patients. Education of patients, medical students, nursing students and staff (see Chapter 2) will help to address the various barriers to effective pain relief (see Box 1.1), and along with the provision of guidelines for simple as well as advanced methods of analgesia, plays an important role in providing the framework for safe and effective pain management. Regular and routine assessment of pain and any side effects of pain relief (see Chapter 3) should be performed and documented, just as a patient's other 'vital signs' – blood pressure, pulse, respiratory rate and temperature – are recorded on a regular basis.

Clinical acute pain management practices should also be based on the best possible evidence available. However, this does not just apply to the drugs and techniques used (see Chapters 4 to 11). Probably more important than the various drugs or analgesic techniques is the need to learn the principles of pain control tailored to the needs of the *individual* patient. There are also some clinical situations or patient groups where pain management may be more problematic and additional knowledge is required (see Chapters 11 to 14).

Adverse effects of undertreated severe acute pain

In the past, many medical and nursing personnel believed that pain was a natural, inevitable, acceptable and harmless consequence of surgery and trauma. However, it is now known that undertreatment of severe acute pain, coupled with the physiological response to surgery known as the stress response, can have a number of adverse consequences (see Box 1.2) and may lead to complications such as myocardial ischemia or infarction and pneumonia. Severe acute pain after surgery may also increase the risk of persistent (chronic) pain.

Box 1.1

Possible barriers to effective pain relief

- A belief that pain is not harmful, or that it is a 'normal' consequence of surgery and injury
- Concerns that pain relief will obscure a surgical diagnosis or mask the signs of surgical complications
- A tendency to underestimate a patient's pain and not recognize the variability in patients' perceptions of pain
- Lack of regular and frequent assessment of pain and any pain-relieving measures
- Fears that the patient will become addicted to opioids
- Concerns about a high risk of respiratory depression with opioids
- Inadequate patient education
- Patient reluctance to request analgesia
- Lack of understanding of the enormous interpatient variability in opioid requirements
- Lack of recognition that age is a better predictor of opioid requirement than weight in the adult patient
- Prolonged dosing intervals and a belief that opioids must not be given more often than every 4 hours
- Insufficient flexibility in dosing schedules (dose and dose intervals)
- Lack of understanding of the need to titrate analgesics to meet the needs of each patient
- Lack of accountability for pain management

Cardiovascular system

Severe pain increases sympathetic nervous system activity and levels of circulating catecholamines, resulting in rises in heart rate, blood pressure and peripheral vascular resistance. These in turn increase the workload of the heart and the oxygen consumption of the myocardium. Myocardial oxygen supply may already be decreased owing to cardiac or respiratory disease, or as a result of hypoxemia from the postoperative pulmonary changes outlined below. If oxygen consumption is greater than oxygen supply, myocardial ischemia (which may be silent in the postoperative period) will result. This may at least partly explain the increased incidence of myocardial ischemia and infarction in the perioperative period.

Increased sympathetic stimulation may also alter regional blood flow, directing blood away from skin and viscera towards brain and heart. Decreased blood flow may impair wound healing and increase muscle spasm.

Severe pain may reduce patient mobility and promote venous stasis. Increases in fibrinogen and platelet activation will increase blood coagulability. Both of these factors will increase the risk of deep vein thrombosis and pulmonary embolism.

Respiratory system

Pain from surgery or injury to the chest or abdomen can exaggerate pulmonary dysfunction, resulting in splinting of the muscles of the diaphragm and chest wall and an impaired ability to cough. This leads to a reduction in lung volumes (vital capacity, forced expiratory volume and functional residual capacity), atelectasis and sputum retention, which can result in hypoxemia and an increased risk of chest infection. Postoperative pulmonary changes are most pronounced on the first or second day after surgery and may take 2 weeks or more to return to preoperative values.

Gastrointestinal and genitourinary systems

Pain can lead to significant delays in gastric emptying and a reduction in intestinal motility. This is thought to be due mainly to activation of a spinal reflex arc and increased sympathetic tone. Other causes of inhibition of motility in the postoperative period include opioid administration and surgery. After abdominal surgery colonic motility is inhibited for 48–72 hours, whereas motility in the stomach and small intestine usually recovers within 12–24 hours. Urinary retention may also occur.

CHAPTER 1

Neuroendocrine and metabolic systems

Pain is believed to play a major part in the activation of the neuroendocrine 'stress response' seen after surgery or trauma which results in the release of a number of hormones (see Box 1.2). This change to a catabolic state of metabolism can lead to hyperglycemia, increases in fibrinogen and platelet activation (increased coagulability), increased protein breakdown and a negative nitrogen balance. Impairments of wound healing and immune function (with a consequent decreased resistance to infection), and sodium and water retention may also occur. The increase in metabolic rate will further increase demands on the cardiorespiratory system.

Box 1.2

Adverse effects of undertreated severe acute pain

Cardiovascular	Tachycardia, hypertension, increased peripheral vascular resistance, increased myocardial oxygen consumption, myocardial ischemia, altered regional blood flow, deep vein thrombosis, pulmonary embolism
Respiratory	Reduced lung volumes, atelectasis, decreased cough, sputum retention, infection, hypoxemia
Gastrointestinal	Decreased gastric and bowel motility, increased risk of bacterial transgression of bowel wall
Genitourinary	Urinary retention
Neuroendocrine/metabolic	Increased catabolic hormones: glucagon, growth hormone, vasopressin, aldosterone, renin and angiotensin
	Reduced anabolic hormones: insulin, testosterone
	This catabolic state leads to hyperglycemia, increased protein breakdown, negative nitrogen balance leading to impaired wound healing and muscle wasting
Musculoskeletal	Muscle spasm, immobility (increasing risk of deep vein thrombosis), muscle wasting leading to prolonged recovery of function
Psychological	Anxiety, fear, helplessness, sleep deprivation, leading to increased pain
Central nervous	Chronic (persistent) pain due to central sensitization

---

Musculoskeletal system

Muscle spasm may reduce respiratory function, and immobility will increase the possibility of venous stasis and deep vein thrombosis. Furthermore, immobility leads to rapid muscle wasting, which can have debilitating functional consequences, in particular in elderly patients.

Psychological effects

Untreated pain can lead to, or increase, patient anxiety, fear, sleeplessness and fatigue. Aggressive or belligerent behavior may be a sign of anxiety and distress. Psychological factors (e.g. anxiety, depression, catastrophizing) and sleep deprivation may also influence the patient's response to pain and pain therapy (see Chapter 3).

Chronic pain

Although in most patients acute pain will resolve over time, there are some who will go on to develop chronic pain after surgery or other injury. It is possible that the risk of developing chronic pain is higher in those patients with severe acute pain (see Chapter 12).

Acute pain management and patient outcomes

Effective analgesia can at least partially reverse some of the harmful effects outlined above and will assist in early mobilization and rehabilitation of the patient. Thus, the treatment of acute pain is important not only for the humanitarian reasons of patient comfort and satisfaction, but also because it may significantly improve outcome by reducing the incidence of postoperative complications and shortening hospital stay, especially in the high-risk patient.

Compared with conventional opioid analgesia (IM, SC or intravenous (IV)), IV PCA (Chapter 8) results in better pain relief and greater patient satisfaction, without increasing the incidence of opioid-related side effects. Epidural analgesia (Chapter 9) has been shown to provide better pain relief than parenteral opioid analgesia and can also decrease the risk of postoperative pulmonary and cardiac complications and allow earlier return of bowel function.

To gain the maximum benefit from pain relief, effective analgesia must be accompanied by an effective postoperative rehabilitation regimen.

References and further reading

Apfelbaum JL, Chen C, Mehta SS et al. (2003) Postoperative pain experience: results from a national survey suggest postoperative pain continues to be under managed. Anesthesia and Analgesia 9: 534–40.

Australian and New Zealand College of Anaesthetists, Faculty of Pain Medicine. Acute Pain Management: Scientific Evidence, 2nd edn. Melbourne: Australian and New Zealand College of Anaesthetists, 2005. Also available online at: *http://www.anzca.edu.au/publications/acutepain.htm* and *http://www7.health.gov.au/nhmrc/publications/synopses/cp104syn.htm*

Bonnet F, Marret E. (2005) Influence of anaesthetic and analgesic techniques on outcome after surgery. British Journal of Anaesthesia 95: 52–8.

Desborough JP. (2000) The stress response to trauma and surgery. British Journal of Anaesthesia 85: 109–17.

Dix P, Sandhar B, Murdoch J et al. (2004) Pain on medical wards in a district general hospital. British Journal of Anaesthesia 92: 235–37.

Dolin SJ, Cashman JN, Bland JM. (2002) Effectiveness of acute postoperative pain management: I. Evidence from published data. British Journal of Anaesthesia 89: 409–23.

International Association for the Study of Pain, European Federation of IASP Chapters. Fact sheet: Unrelieved pain is a major global healthcare problem. 2004. Available online at: *http://www.painreliefhumanright.com/pdf/04a_global_day_fact_sheet.pdf*

Miaskowski C, Crews J, Ready LB et al. (1999) Anesthesia-based pain services improve the quality of postoperative pain management. Pain 80: 23–9.

Moss E, Taverner T, Norton R et al. (2005) A survey of postoperative pain management in fourteen hospitals in the UK. Acute Pain 7: 13–20.

Rocchi A, Chung F, Forte L. (2002) Canadian survey of postsurgical pain and pain medication experiences. Canadian Journal of Anesthesia. 49: 1053–6.

Whelan CT, Jin L, Meltzer D. (2004) Pain and satisfaction with pain control in hospitalized medical patients: no such thing as low risk. Archives of Internal Medicine 164: 175–80.

Organizational considerations

As noted in Chapter 1, acute pain relief for many patients remains suboptimal, despite the advances of the past 10–20 years that have seen the widespread introduction of new analgesic techniques and drugs. One of the reasons for continued inadequate treatment may be that it is probably a case not so much of 'what is used' but rather of 'how it is used'.

To a large extent this will depend on the systems involved in the delivery of pain relief. Even 'simple' methods (e.g. oral administration of an opioid) can be made much more effective if proper consideration is given to aspects of the delivery that are not related to either the technique or the drug used, but rather to staff and patient education and the systems that institutions have in place to provide patients with safe and effective analgesia.

Education of all staff and patients will play a key role in improving pain relief. However, the provision of guidelines and standardization for 'simple' as well as more advanced analgesic techniques will also help. Regular patient assessment is also vital (see Chapter 3), as is the correct response to inadequate pain relief or the onset of any side effects of treatment. Although some institutions will have acute pain services others will not, but the principles of effective and safe acute pain management remain the same.

CHAPTER 2

Education

One of the best-recognized reasons for past and current deficiencies in the management of acute pain is inadequate education of medical, nursing and allied health staff and students, patients, and their families and friends. Inadequate knowledge, misconceptions and the persistence of some of the myths that surround pain management continue to result in barriers that prevent optimal analgesia in many patients (see Chapter 1).

Better education of all groups is needed if more sophisticated methods of pain relief (such as patient-controlled and epidural analgesia) are to be managed safely and effectively, and if better results are to be gained from conventional methods of pain relief.

Medical staff

Education of junior medical staff should include all aspects of the management of acute pain. In particular, they must be aware of the detrimental effects that unrelieved pain can have on patient wellbeing and outcome after trauma and surgery (see Chapter 1). Although they will not be directly responsible for more advanced, newer methods of pain relief, they must have a sound working knowledge of them. They must be aware of possible complications and drug interactions, and be able to explain the techniques to both patients and their relatives. Responsibility for more conventional methods of analgesia is often delegated to junior medical staff. A better understanding of how to use the various drugs and techniques available will help to improve the effectiveness of these forms of pain relief.

Nursing staff

Ward nurses are directly involved in the management of all forms of pain relief and play a key role in ensuring that analgesia, whether simple or sophisticated, is safely and effectively managed. Education and accreditation programs are therefore essential. The education requirements are twofold – general and specialized.

General education will lead to a better practical understanding of the relevance of appropriate pain relief for patient wellbeing and outcome, as well as the drugs and techniques used (including simple techniques). Important topics include early recognition and treatment of side effects, the physiological and psychological benefits of better acute pain management, and the importance of patient education. The appropriate use of non-pharmacological measures should be understood, as well as issues arising from the treatment of pain in cognitively impaired patients and in patients from different cultures.

The time available for education in a hospital is often limited. Priorities must therefore be set regarding the importance of various pain topics. It is much more important for nurses to realize that the best measure of pain intensity is the patient's self-report, and to understand the principles of opioid titration based on this self-report, than for them to be taught excessive detail about individual drugs or the physiology of pain.

Specialized education may then lead to a better understanding of more sophisticated methods of pain relief, such as patient-controlled analgesia (PCA), and epidural or other regional analgesia.

Many institutions require some form of certification or accreditation before nurses can assume responsibility for a patient whose pain is being managed using one of the more advanced methods of pain relief listed above. Accreditation programs often consist of:

- verbal and written information (e.g. lectures or workshops and booklets);
- written assessment (e.g. multiple choice questionnaires);
- practical assessment (e.g. demonstration of ability to program machines, administer epidural bolus doses).

Reaccreditation every 1–2 years will help ensure that knowledge and practices are regularly updated. Formal education programs need to be supplemented with informal 'one-on-one' teaching in the ward.

Patients

Many patients still rate the fear of pain as a major preoperative concern (along with nausea and vomiting), and many still expect significant pain after surgery. Their attitudes and expectations can affect pain perception and analgesic requirements.

Patients who learn to assess their pain, and who are made aware that they should ask for more pain relief when needed, will have more control over the dose and delivery of analgesic drugs, regardless of the analgesic technique used. Appropriate education and information can therefore be a powerful tool in helping to ensure effective pain relief.

Information should be given to each patient and tailored to their needs. It should include both *procedural* and *sensory* information (see below). Adequate education and information can lead to a reduction in anxiety, analgesic use and perceptions of pain intensity.

Information can be presented in a number of ways: verbally, in a booklet, or on a video. In general, a mix of these methods probably gives the best results. Examples of patient information available on the internet and in printed form are given in the Appendices at the end of this chapter. Although education about pain management should ideally start before it is needed, this will not always be possible (e.g. after an emergency operation or trauma).

It is known that most patients remember only a small part of any information presented at one time. Therefore, it will need to be repeated a number of times, including during treatment.

General education

Patients should be made aware of a number of general factors important to their pain relief. These include the following.

Treatment goals and benefits

Patients should know why effective analgesia is important for their recovery as well as their comfort. The benefits of physiotherapy and early mobilization should be explained. They should be assured that every attempt will be made to make them as comfortable as possible, but that pain scores of zero at all times are usually not achievable with medications currently available. Patients should be aware that it is better to treat pain early than to delay until it is severe.

Options available for the treatment of acute pain

Options for the treatment of acute pain will vary from case to case, but patients should play an active role in expressing their preference after the possible risks, benefits and side effects have been explained.

Monitoring pain and its treatment

Methods used in the measurement of pain should be outlined. Patients should know that there is no 'right or wrong' answer for pain scores, as these reflect their own subjective experience, but that these scores are helpful for tailoring their analgesic requirements. In some patients it may be helpful to explain that excessive sedation means they need a little less opioid.

The need to communicate inadequate analgesia or side effects

Patients should be encouraged to tell their doctors and nurses if analgesia is inadequate, or if they are experiencing side effects. If intermittent opioid regimens are being used, the importance of asking for the next dose as soon as they begin to feel uncomfortable should be explained. They should not feel they are 'bothering' busy nursing or medical staff.

Concerns about the risks of addiction

Many patients (or their relatives) are still concerned about the risks of addiction, dependence or tolerance to opioids. Repeated explanations may be required to allay these fears.

Specialized education

Explanations of individual analgesic techniques such as PCA and epidural analgesia should be given, including the expected duration of therapy and subsequent analgesic management. The description of PCA does not have to be technically detailed. However, patients must know that they can press the button whenever they are uncomfortable, and that they are the only ones allowed to do this (i.e. family and staff are not permitted to do so). They need also to understand that PCA, when correctly used, is an inherently safe technique. Patients should be assured that, despite the use of these techniques, direct personal contact time with nursing staff will not be reduced.

The safety of PCA and 'being in control' must be emphasized. Most of the complications of PCA therapy will be due to the opioids, although an explanation of other causes of some side effects may be useful. For example, a patient experiencing nausea or vomiting after bowel surgery may be reluctant to use PCA if they are told that the only cause of this is the opioid.

The possible side effects and complications of epidural analgesia also should be explained, including the need to report to the hospital immediately if increasing back pain or neurological symptoms occur at any time before or after discharge from hospital.

Standardization

'Standard' orders and guidelines are commonly used for some of the more advanced methods of pain relief, such as PCA and epidural analgesia (see Chapters 8 and 9). However, standardization may also help to make traditional methods of pain relief safer and more effective. This may be as simple as a statement suggesting that 'paracetamol should be ordered on a regular basis for all patients unless contraindicated', or more complex, such as the provision of guidelines for intermittent IV, SC or oral administration of opioids (see examples in Chapter 7).

Consideration should be given to standardizing the following aspects of pain relief, regardless of the drug or technique used, and of whether the analgesia is considered 'simple' or 'advanced':

- Education – nursing, medical and patient
- Drugs used – analgesic and non-analgesic (e.g. for the treatment of nausea and vomiting)

- Drug doses and concentrations
- Non-drug treatment (e.g. supplemental oxygen)
- Monitoring requirements (regular assessments of adequacy of analgesia and adverse effects)
- The response to inadequate analgesia
- The response to and treatment of side effects
- Nursing procedures
- Equipment used.

As with all guidelines, the aim is to try and improve the quality of clinical decision-making and reduce unnecessary variations in clinical practice, not to dictate practice.

Acute pain services

The first anesthesiologist-based acute pain service (APS) in the USA was started by Ready in 1986. Since that time many hospitals worldwide have followed suit, and the number continues to grow.

There has been some debate as to the best form of acute pain service. Currently, structures vary from nurse-based, anesthesiologist-led but without daily participation by an anesthesiologist, to anesthesiologist-based (usually run by anesthesiologists because the knowledge required and techniques used are similar to those used in anesthesia). All rely on APS nurses and, regardless of the model chosen, an organized team approach is important. Whether simple or 'high-tech' analgesic options are used, patients whose pain relief is managed by an APS may have less pain, suffer fewer side effects and express greater satisfaction than those whose pain management is supervised by less experienced staff.

The nurse-based, anesthesiologist-supervised model described by Rawal (1997) seeks to involve all nurses in the provision of better analgesia, regardless of the technique used. They propose that improved education and regular monitoring of pain and pain relief ('making pain visible') will lead to better analgesia for all patients. There are also significant advantages in terms of cost.

Unfortunately, some anesthesiologist-based APS have tended to concentrate on the 'high-tech' approaches and placed much less emphasis on improving the simple methods of pain relief throughout their hospital. This benefits only a small proportion of patients. This need not be the case, as the organization of an APS can be such that pain management for all patients in the institution will improve. As with the nurse-based service, an anesthesiologist-based APS should assist in the development of undergraduate and postgraduate education programs and better protocols for all analgesic techniques used throughout the hospital (Box 2.1).

Box 2.1

Role of an acute pain service

1. Education (initial, updates)
- anesthesiologists
- nurses (accreditation/reaccreditation programs)
- patients and carers/families
- medical and nursing students
- junior medical staff
- surgeons and physicians
- pharmacists
- physiotherapists
- hospital administrators
- health insurance carriers

2. Introduction and supervision of more advanced analgesic techniques including:
- patient-controlled analgesia
- epidural and intrathecal analgesia
- other continuous regional analgesia techniques

3. Assistance in improving traditional analgesic treatment regimens, including:
- intermittent opioid regimens (IM, SC, IV and oral)
- non-opioid analgesia

4. Standardization of:
- equipment
- 'standard orders' for advanced analgesic techniques
  - drugs, doses and drug dilutions
  - diagnosis and treatment of side effects
  - specific monitoring requirements for each analgesic technique
- nursing procedure protocols
- guidelines for the monitoring of all patients receiving opioids
- guidelines for the use of other analgesic drugs and adjuvant agents
- non-drug treatment orders, e.g. use of oxygen, use of antireflux valves

5. 24-hour availability of pain service personnel
- for scheduled daily rounds of all patients under care of the APS
- for additional reviews as needed of patients with ongoing pain problems
- for treatment of complications of pain treatment
- for initiation of new pain management modalities on request
- for advice about any pain management problems

6. Collaboration and communication with other medical and nursing services including:
- – chronic pain clinics
- – drug and alcohol services
- – palliative care services
- – surgical services

7. Regular audit of activity and continuous quality improvement

8. Clinical research

Anesthesiologist-based services may also have other advantages. The APS anesthesiologists will have expert knowledge about the pharmacology of all analgesic agents, the different delivery techniques available, and the risks and benefits of those techniques. They may therefore be more likely to tailor 'standard' orders to suit individual patients. They will also have a good understanding of the disease processes of the patients they are seeing, and may be called on to help with acute postoperative and other medical problems.

Key points

Evidence level

II Preoperative education improves patient or carer knowledge of pain and encourages a more positive attitude towards pain relief

III Implementation of an acute pain service may improve pain relief and reduce the incidence of side effects

III Staff education and the use of guidelines improve pain assessment, pain relief and prescribing practices

III Even 'simple' techniques of pain relief can be more effective if attention is given to education, documentation, patient assessment and the provision of appropriate guidelines and policies

Clinical practice points

Successful management of acute pain requires close liaison with all personnel involved in the care of the patient

More effective acute pain management will result from appropriate education and organizational structures for the delivery of pain relief rather than the analgesic techniques themselves

Reproduced with permission from Acute Pain Management: Scientific Evidence ANZCA and FPM (2005)

References and further reading

American Society of Anesthesiologists. (2004) Practice guidelines for acute pain management in the perioperative setting. American Society of Anesthesiologists. Anesthesiology 100: 1573–81.

Australian and New Zealand College of Anaesthetists, Faculty of Pain Medicine. Acute Pain Management: Scientific Evidence, 2nd edn. Melbourne: Australian and New Zealand College of Anaesthetists, 2005. Also available online at: *http://www.anzca.edu.au/publications/acutepain.htm* and *http://www7.health.gov.au/nhmrc/publications/synopses/cp104syn.htm*

Bardiau FM, Taviaux NF, Albert A et al. (2003) An intervention study to enhance postoperative pain management. Anesthesia and Analgesia 96: 179–85.

Breivik H. (2002) How to implement an acute pain service. Best Practice and Research in Clinical Anaesthesiology 16: 527–47.

Macintyre PE, Runciman WBR, Webb RK. (1990) An acute pain service in an Australian teaching hospital – the first year. Medical Journal of Australia 153: 417–20.

McDonnell A, Nicholl J, Read SM. (2003) Acute pain teams and the management of postoperative pain: a systematic review and meta-analysis. Journal of Advanced Nursing 4: 261–73.

Miaskowski C, Crews J, Ready LB et al. (1999) Anesthesia-based pain services improve the quality of postoperative pain management. Pain 80: 23–9.

Moss E, Taverner T, Norton R et al. (2005) A survey of postoperative pain management in fourteen hospitals in the UK. Acute Pain 7: 13–20.

Powell AE, Davies HT, Bannister J et al. (2004) Rhetoric and reality on acute pain services in the UK: a national postal questionnaire survey. British Journal of Anaesthesia 92: 689–93.

Rawal N. (1997) Organization of acute pain services: a low cost model. Acta Anaesthiologica Scandinavica 111: 188–90.

Rawal N. (2005) Organization, function, and implementation of acute pain service. Anesthesiology Clinics of North America 23: 211–25.

Ready L.B, Oden R, Chadwick HS et al. (1988) Development of an anesthesiology-based postoperative pain management service. Anesthesiology 68: 100–106.

Roth W, Kling J, Gockel I et al. (2005) Dissatisfaction with postoperative pain management – a prospective analysis of 1071 patients. Acute Pain 7: 75–83.

Schug SA, Harida RP. (1993) Development and organizational structure of an acute pain service in a major teaching hospital. Australian New Zealand Journal of Surgery 63: 8–13.

Schug SA, Torrie JJ. (1993) Safety assessment of postoperative pain management by an acute pain service. Pain 55: 389–91.

Shapiro A, Zohar E, Kantor M et al. (2003) Establishing a nurse-based anaesthesiologist-supervised inpatient acute pain service: experience of 4,617 patients. Journal of Clinical Anesthesia 16: 415–20.

Stadler M, Schlander M, Braeckman M et al. (2004) A cost–utility and cost–effectiveness analysis of an acute pain service. Journal of Clinical Anesthesia 16: 159–67.

Story DA, Shelton AC, Poustie SJ et al. (2006) Effect of an anaesthesia department-led critical care outreach and acute pain service on postoperative serious adverse events. Anaesthesia 61: 24–8.

Werner MU, Søholm L, Rotbøll-Nielsen P et al. (2002) Does an acute pain service improve postoperative outcome? Anesthesia and Analgesia 95: 1361–72.

Wheatley RJ, Madej TH, Jackson IJB, Hunter D. (1991) The first year's experience of an acute pain service. British Journal of Anaesthesia 67: 353–9.

Wheatley RG, Madej TH. (2003) Organization of an acute pain service. In: Rowbotham DJ, Macintyre PE, eds. Clinical pain management: acute pain. London: Arnold.

Appendix 2A

Examples of patient information available on the internet

Australian and New Zealand College of Anaesthetists, Faculty of Pain Medicine

Managing acute pain: a guide for patients. http: //www.anzca.edu.au/ publications/acutepain.htm

Royal College of Anaesthetists

- *Epidurals for pain relief after surgery. http: //www.rcoa.ac.uk/docs/eprs. pdf*
- *Nerve damage associated with a spinal or epidural injection. http: //www. rcoa.ac.uk/docs/nerve–spinal.pdf*

Appendix 2B

Example of printed patient information sheets

Acute Pain Service, Royal Adelaide Hospital

PCA and epidural analgesia – information for patients.

Acute Pain Service, Royal Perth Hospital

Letter given to patients who have had epidural analgesia on discharge from hospital.

Both reproduced with permission.

Appendix 2A: Royal Adelaide Hospital

Acute Pain Service Department of Anaesthesia

Patient guide to patient-controlled analgesia and epidural analgesia

There is more information about the general management of acute pain in the information sheet about anaesthesia. Please read this as well as the information in this pamphlet.

For the treatment of some types of acute pain you may be offered a more advanced method of pain relief. Here at the Royal Adelaide Hospital the two most commonly used of these methods are *patient-controlled analgesia* and *epidural analgesia*.

If you have one of these forms of pain relief you will be seen at least once a day by an anaesthetist and nurse from the *Acute Pain Service* (APS) in addition to the doctors and nurses on your ward. The APS is part of the Department of Anaesthesia at the Royal Adelaide Hospital. Anaesthetists are the doctors who look after you during your anaesthetic, but they also specialize in pain relief. The APS also has an anaesthetist on call 24 hours a day to help with pain control.

Patient-controlled analgesia

Patient-controlled analgesia (or PCA for short) means that you have control over your own pain relief. A machine called a PCA pump can be used to give you a small dose of a strong pain-relieving drug such as morphine or fentanyl. Usually this machine will be attached to the drip (intravenous line or IV) in your arm. If you are uncomfortable, you press a button and the machine will pump a small dose of the drug into your drip. You can do this whenever you are uncomfortable – you do not need to tell the nurse first. The amount of pain medicine delivered by the machine each time you press the button, as well as other settings on the machine, will be ordered by the anaesthetist from the APS. The PCA machine will be programmed by your nurse according to these orders.

How often can I press the button?

You can press the PCA button whenever you feel uncomfortable. However, once the button has been pushed and the PCA machine has delivered the dose, built-in timers in the machine will 'lock out' further pushes for 5 minutes. This means that if you push the button within this time, the PCA machine will not deliver another dose.

This is so that you have time to feel the effect of one dose of pain-relieving drug before getting another dose. Remember, the aim is to make you comfortable – it is not always possible to be completely pain free.

Who is allowed to press the PCA button?

The patient is the ONLY person allowed to press the button. Do not allow ANY hospital staff, relatives or friends to do so.

Will the pain-relieving drug work immediately?

No. These drugs need to get to the brain and spinal cord, so it may take 5 minutes or longer to get the full effect. If you are about to do something that you know will hurt, like coughing or moving, press the PCA button about 5 minutes *before* doing it.

What if the pain medicine doesn't work?

If you are pressing the PCA button quite frequently and are still uncomfortable, tell your nurse. They will first check that the IV is running properly. As long as you are not having problems staying awake, your nurse may increase the amount of pain medicine you get when you press the button. If necessary, your nurse will contact the APS.

Can I overdose?

PCA is probably one of the safest ways of giving strong pain-relieving medicines. The dose that you get with each press of the button is very small. If you were getting just a little too much you would feel sleepy. This means that you would not press the button again. Your nurse would also notice this and would reduce the amount of drug delivered with each push of the button and, if necessary, treat the sleepiness.

How long will I use PCA for?

When your doctors on the ward allow you to drink it means that your IV may soon be removed. PCA will usually stop at this time. You will be ordered other pain-relieving medicines should you need them.

Epidural analgesia

Epidural analgesia is often used to treat pain during childbirth. It can also be used to treat acute pain after some operations and accidents. Most pain-relieving medicines work by acting on the brain and spinal cord. They are usually carried there in the bloodstream. With epidural analgesia, the pain-relieving drugs can be placed much closer to where they are needed, near the spinal cord.

You would often have epidural analgesia for pain relief after your surgery if you also had it during your surgery. This means it would be started by an anaesthetist, usually at the time of the operation. The anaesthetist would insert a needle in your back into a space called the *epidural space*. A very small and soft plastic tube is then threaded through the needle and the needle is removed. This plastic tube is called the *epidural catheter*. The epidural catheter is fixed to the skin on your back with tape. It is then connected to a machine which slowly pumps the pain-relieving medicines into the epidural space. From here it is easy for the pain medicines to get to the spinal cord and nerves.

What are the advantages of epidural analgesia?

Epidural analgesia can give the best pain relief of all, but is not necessary after all operations or accidents. We think that it is most likely to be good for patients who are elderly or have major medical problems, or who are having very major surgery. In these patients very good pain relief may reduce the risk of complications after surgery.

What are the risks of epidural analgesia?

Complications occasionally occur. Most of these are minor and easily treated. More serious complications may occur, but these are extremely rare. Some of the possible complications are:

- The epidural does not work or does not work properly. If this happens and the anaesthetists can't help make it work, you will be given another kind of pain relief.
- There can be an infection at the site where the epidural catheter goes through your skin. This may be a little red and sore for a few days, but usually goes away without needing treatment. The APS will see you every day until it is healing.
- Your blood pressure may fall. However, after surgery this usually happens when you are also a little dehydrated, and it is often a sign that you need more fluid.
- You may get a headache. Sometimes this can happen if the needle that is used to place the epidural catheter goes past the epidural space. Most often, however, any headache that you get after your surgery is likely to be due to another cause. If the headache worries you let your nurse know and they can contact the APS.
- Nerve damage can occur rarely and in most cases this heals within a few weeks or months.

- Very rarely an abscess or blood clot can occur in the epidural space. It is difficult to get a good idea of risk, but it may be between 1 in every 10 000 to 150 000 patients. If the abscess or blood clot was big enough to press on the spinal cord then permanent nerve damage or paraplegia could occur, especially if treatment is not started as soon as possible. At the Royal Adelaide Hospital the APS and the nurses on the ward are aware of the risk, even though it is very rare. The regular monitoring that we use is designed to pick up complications at an early stage. We also have strict protocols for looking after epidural analgesia that we believe may lower the risk of these complications.

What pain-relieving drugs are used with epidural analgesia?

We often use a mixture of local anaesthetic and fentanyl (a morphine-like pain medicine) or just local anaesthetic by itself.

Can I move around or walk when I have epidural analgesia?

Yes. It is important to move around after surgery. When your surgeon says you can get out of bed or walk, it is important that you do this as well. This can help reduce the risk of chest infections or blood clots in your legs. You can walk with an epidural catheter in your back. However, you should ask your nurse before starting. At first, you will walk with two nurses, just to make sure that you don't faint or lose your balance. When you get out of bed do it very slowly, just in case you become dizzy.

What if the epidural analgesia doesn't work?

If you are uncomfortable tell your nurse, who will check the epidural catheter. They may increase the amount of pain medicine that you are getting, or give you an extra dose. If necessary, the APS may also be contacted.

Will my legs feel numb, weak or heavy?

If you are having an operation, the epidural will often be used as part of the anaesthetic as well as for pain relief afterwards. A strong local anaesthetic may be given during the operation. This means that your legs may feel numb and heavy immediately after the operation. This will wear off in a few hours. The local anaesthetics that we use for epidural analgesia after the operation will not be as strong, so your legs should feel virtually normal. When you are back in your ward your nurse will regularly ask you if you have any numbness anywhere, or if your legs feel weak. They will also ask you to lift your knee up to your chest.

If you notice any numbness or weakness, let your nurse or doctor know straight away. The aim is to keep you comfortable but still able to move around in bed, sit out of bed and even walk, when your doctors allow it.

Will my legs be numb, weak or heavy when I leave hospital?

No. *We need to know if this happens,* even if you had your epidural weeks ago. In the unlikely event that you have gone home and noticed any numbness, heaviness or weakness in your legs, or have trouble passing water, or have a pain in your back that is getting worse, *you should immediately phone the Royal Adelaide Hospital and ask to speak to the anaesthetist on duty for the APS.* The phone number is **08 8222 4000.**

Appendix 2B: Royal Perth Hospital
Department of Anaesthesia & Pain Medicine

You have had an *epidural infusion* while in hospital. While this provides excellent pain relief and aids recovery after surgery, there is a minimal risk of serious but rare complications, including bleeding or infection around the spinal cord. These may be delayed in presentation.

If you experience in the next days or weeks:

* new severe back pain
* new weakness, increasing numbness or new loss of sensation in your legs
* new loss of bladder or bowel control,

consult your GP or an Emergency Department immediately. Please show this card to the treating doctor.

In case of concern, please phone Royal Perth Hospital on 9224 2244 and ask to speak to the Pain Registrar on Page 6450.

Professor SA Schug
Director, Pain Medicine

3 Assessment of the patient with acute pain

Chapter contents

Effective and safe management of acute pain is best achieved by tailoring pain therapies to the individual patient. This means that the appropriate treatment regimen must be selected and then modified as needed, based on assessments of the adequacy of pain relief and the onset of any adverse effects or complications.

In recent years, increasing emphasis has been placed on the need to assess pain on a regular basis – pain as 'the 5th vital sign' (JCAHO, 2001) – often using pain scores. Less emphasis, however, has been placed on the need to monitor for the early onset of significant side effects related to treatment (e.g. opioid-induced respiratory depression) or potentially disastrous complications (e.g. permanent paraplegia associated with epidural analgesia). Without such monitoring, safe management of acute pain is not possible.

In the chapters that follow, suggested strategies for the optimal use of many of the drugs and techniques used in acute pain management are outlined, as are some of the various side effects and complications that may result from their use. The basic tools that will allow pain and the response to therapy to be assessed, and the appropriate treatment regimens to be selected and then altered to suit individual patients, are described below.

Assessment of pain and pain relief

The International Association for the Study of Pain (IASP) defines pain as 'An unpleasant sensory and emotional experience associated with actual or potential tissue damage or described in terms of such damage' (Merskey, 1979).

Pain is therefore a very individual and subjective experience. There are a host of behavioral, psychological and social factors that may increase or decrease the patient's response to, and report of, pain. They may include previous pain experiences, cultural background, social supports, the meaning and consequences of the pain (e.g. disease or surgical prognosis, loss of employment), coping styles, the degree of control felt over the pain and disease, and fear, anxiety or depression. These will interact to produce what the patient then describes as pain. Pain is therefore different from nociception (see below).

The type of pain may also affect the choice of treatment regimen and the response to analgesic therapies. Pain can be broadly classified into two main types, nociceptive and neuropathic, although both may be present in the same patient at the same time. Common clinical features of the different pain types are summarized in Box 3.1.

Nociceptive pain (somatic or visceral) is the most common type of pain seen in acute clinical settings. It results from the stimulation of specialized sensory nerve endings called nociceptors, as a consequence of tissue damage or inflammation (e.g. after surgery, infection or trauma). Intense and ongoing peripheral nociceptive stimuli will increase the excitability of neurons in the spinal cord, leading to central sensitization. Peripheral and central sensitization result in the amplification of subsequent pain stimuli (both in intensity and area of pain) and a lowered pain threshold.

Neuropathic pain is associated with injury or disease of the peripheral or central nervous system. Following such injury a number of changes occur, including the development of central sensitization, reorganization of synaptic connections in the spinal cord, and hyperexcitability of damaged peripheral nerves. As a result, the patient may exhibit signs and symptoms that are typical of neuropathic pain (Box 3.1). Neuropathic pain is a common cause of chronic symptoms, but can also be a component of acute pain (e.g. following surgery or trauma) – see Chapter 12.

The key components of assessment are the pain history and measures of pain severity and/or response to treatment. There also needs to be an understanding of some of the psychological factors that may contribute to the reported pain experience.

Box 3.1

Nociceptive and neuropathic pain

Pain type	Clinical features may include
Nociceptive pain	
Somatic	Sharp, hot or stinging pain which is usually well localized to the area of injury
Visceral	Dull, cramping, or colicky pain which is often poorly localized
	Pain may be referred over a wide area
	There may be associated symptoms such as nausea and sweating
Neuropathic pain	History of injury or disease leading to damage to the peripheral or central nervous system, e.g. brachial plexus avulsion, amputation of a limb, spinal cord injury, acute herpes zoster (shingles), stroke
	Evidence of damage to peripheral or central nervous system, including spinal cord (sensory loss, motor weakness, bowel or bladder sphincter abnormalities, reflex changes)
	Pain in an area of sensory loss (but not necessarily confined to this area)
	Increased sympathetic activity (alterations in skin color, temperature and texture, sweating)
	Pain that is different in nature from nociceptive pain, e.g. burning, shooting or stabbing pain
	Pain may be spontaneous or paroxysmal
	Pain that appears to be responding poorly to opioids
	Phantom phenomenon
	Allodynia: the sensation of pain in response to a stimulus that does not normally cause pain (e.g. light touch)
	Hyperalgesia: an increased (i.e. exaggerated) response to a stimulus that is normally painful
	Dysesthesias: unpleasant abnormal sensations

Pain history

A pain history, in addition to a general medical history and examination, provides important information that will help in the diagnosis of both the pain state (cause and type of pain) and the response to treatment. It also allows an assessment of the many behavioral, psychological and social factors that might play a part in the patient's pain experience. The basic elements of a pain history are summarized in Box 3.2.

A pain history should not only be taken when the patient is first seen, but repeated whenever there is a change in the nature or intensity of the pain, or when the pain is not responding well to treatment.

Box 3.2

Basic elements of a pain history

Site of pain	Primary location and any radiation
Conditions associated with pain onset	e.g. time of onset, precipitating events
Character of the pain	e.g. sharp, dull, colicky, throbbing, aching, burning, shooting
Intensity of the pain	At rest and on movement
	Duration
	Whether continuous or intermittent
	Any aggravating or relieving factors
Associated symptoms	e.g. nausea, sweating
Function	Effect of pain on mobility, activities and sleep
Current and prior treatments for pain	Doses of analgesic drugs, frequency of use, efficacy, side effects
Relevant medical history	Prior or coexisting medical and pain conditions and treatment outcomes
Other patient factors	Beliefs concerning the cause of the pain
	Knowledge, expectations and preferences for pain management
	Expectations of outcome of pain treatment
	Typical coping response for stress or pain, including the presence of anxiety or psychiatric disorders (e.g. depression or psychosis)
	Expectations and beliefs about pain, stress and postoperative course

Adapted from Acute Pain Management: Scientific Evidence ANZCA and FPM 2005

Measurement

There are a number of simple clinical techniques for the assessment and measurement of pain and its response to treatment. Given the multidimensional nature of the pain experience, it is not surprising that there is often a poor correlation between the patient's assessment of pain and the nursing or medical staff's estimate of the pain that patient is experiencing. The best pain measures involve self-reporting by the patient rather than observer assessment.

Assessment of function is also important, especially if a patient is unable to give a self-report of pain, when functional assessment may be less biased than observation of behavior and/or vital signs.

Unidimensional measures

In adults, three common self-reporting methods used to measure pain intensity (a single dimension of pain) are the visual analog scale (VAS), the verbal numerical rating scale (VNRS) and the verbal descriptor scale (VDS). Each of these is reasonably reliable as long as any endpoints and adjectives employed are carefully selected and standardized. Although they are often used to compare levels of pain between patients, these methods of scoring are probably of most use as measures of change in the level of pain within each patient and the effectiveness of treatment of that pain.

Visual analog scale

The VAS uses a 10 cm line with endpoint descriptors such as 'no pain' marked at the left-hand end of the line and 'worst pain imaginable' marked at the right-hand end. There are no other cues marked on the line. The patient is asked to mark a point on the line that best represents their pain. The distance from 'no pain' to the patient's mark is then measured in millimeters – this is the VAS score (1–100).

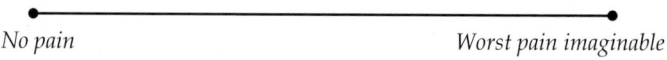

No pain   *Worst pain imaginable*

To simplify these measurements, VAS slide rules have been developed. On the front of the slide rule is a 10 cm line with the endpoints such as 'no pain' and 'worst pain imaginable'. The reverse side shows the same line marked at millimeter intervals. The patient moves the slide along the line on the front of the rule to the point that best represents the pain. The corresponding VAS measurement is then read off the back of the rule.

The disadvantages of the VAS system are that it can be more time-consuming than other simple scoring methods, specific equipment is needed (albeit very simple), and some patients may have difficulty understanding or performing this score, especially in the immediate postoperative period. One advantage of the method is that the wording can be written in many different languages.

The VAS scale can also be adapted to measure other variables, such as patient satisfaction, side effects such as nausea and vomiting, and degree of pain relief. The endpoints of a VAS measuring pain relief would be 'no relief' and 'complete relief'.

Verbal numerical rating scale

The VNRS is similar to the VAS. Patients are asked to imagine that '0 equals no pain' and '10 equals the worst pain imaginable', and then to give a number on this scale that would best represent their pain. Similarly, they could be asked to imagine that '0 equals no pain relief' and '10 equals complete relief of pain'. The advantage of this type of system is that it does not require any equipment. However, problems may occur if there is a language barrier or the patient has some other difficulty in understanding the scoring system.

There is a good correlation between the VAS and VNRS.

Verbal descriptor scale

Verbal descriptor scales use different words to rate the severity of pain, such as none, mild, moderate, severe and excruciating. These scales are quick and easy to use and may be more reliable in some patients, e.g. the elderly. A VDS can also be used to measure pain relief with words such as none, slight, moderate, good and complete.

What pain score is 'comfortable'?

It is usually not possible, practical or safe to aim for complete pain relief at all times with most of the drugs and drug administration techniques currently used in the treatment of acute pain. The aim of treatment should be patient comfort, both at rest and with physical activity such as coughing or ambulation.

Just as pain is a very individual experience, the correlation of 'comfort' and a specific pain score may show marked interpatient variability. Therefore, alterations in analgesic regimens may need to take into account a number of factors, such as the patient's pain score, the level they would regard as comfortable, and their functional ability. The presence or absence of any side effects from analgesic drugs will also affect what alterations are made to treatment orders. Alterations based solely on a particular pain score may lead to excessive treatment in some patients, and to under-treatment in others.

Coping styles may also affect self-reports of pain and the ability to tolerate pain. Discrepancies between pain behavior and a patient's self- report of pain may result from different coping skills. Staff should not necessarily assume, for example, that a patient who is smiling, reading or sleeping is comfortable.

Similarly, high pain scores may not always require the dose of an analgesic to be increased. This does not mean that the patient's report of pain is disbelieved, but that the appropriate therapeutic response to the reported pain may vary between patients. For example, patients who are very anxious may report high pain levels (see below), yet treatment (not necessarily drug treatment) of that anxiety, rather than an automatic increase in analgesic dose, may be preferable. Other patients may have pain which is not always responsive to opioid drugs and which may require treatment using other classes of analgesics (e.g. neuropathic pain).

When should pain be assessed?

Patients are usually asked to rate their pain when they are resting. However, a better indicator of the effectiveness of analgesia is an assessment of the pain caused by physical activity, such as coughing, deep breathing or movement. Therefore, pain scores at rest and with movement or coughing should be recorded.

Pain should be reassessed regularly during the treatment period; the frequency of this assessment will vary according to the analgesic regimen chosen and the patient's response to therapy. The frequency of assessment should be increased if the pain is poorly controlled, or if the pain stimulus or treatment interventions are changing. A repeat pain history will help determine whether the nature of the pain has changed, if there is a new cause for the pain (e.g. postoperative complication), or whether a change should be made to the analgesic regimen.

Assessment of function

Measurement of pain is only one part of the assessment of adequacy of analgesia. Assessment of function – for example the ability to take deep breaths, cough, ambulate and cooperate with physiotherapy after surgery – gives an important indication of the effectiveness of analgesic therapy. An analgesic regimen should not be presumed to have 'failed' solely on the basis of reported high pain scores, as there may be many reasons for this (see later). However, functional limitation as a result of pain means that re-evaluation of therapy is required.

Other measures of pain

In some patients it may not be possible to obtain reliable self-reports of pain (e.g. where there are problems with communication due to language difficulties or cognitive impairment). In such cases alternative measures of pain will be needed, such as assessment of patient behaviors (e.g. grimacing, groaning, guarding or rubbing).

At times, discrepancies between a patient's behavior and their self-report of pain may result from differences in psychological, social and cultural factors that can modulate the amount of pain experienced and reported. In elderly patients (see Chapter 14) a good correlation has been shown between unidimensional and behavioral measures in those who are cognitively intact, but it is not known whether the same correlation exists in those with cognitive impairment.

Assessment of pain by observing patient behavior and/or vital signs should therefore be reserved only for situations when self-report measures cannot be used.

Patient satisfaction

Assessments of patient satisfaction are often used as an indicator of 'good' or 'bad' pain relief. However, they are really more a measure of the patient's overall satisfaction with their treatment. They can be influenced by factors other than the degree of pain, such as their expectations of pain, interference with functioning, analgesia-related adverse effects, and their relationship with medical and nursing staff (e.g. ability to communicate well, kindness and care shown, and information given). Patients may report high levels of satisfaction even though they have moderate to severe acute pain.

Psychological factors

As outlined earlier, pain is an individual and subjective experience to which psychological and social factors contribute. That is, the intensity of acute pain perceived and a number of psychological, behavioral, environmental and social factors may influence the patient's response to pain and pain therapy. These factors are important in acute as well as chronic pain settings, and in the transition from acute to chronic pain.

Preoperative anxiety, depression and neuroticism may all be associated with reports of higher pain intensities after surgery. Catastrophizing is also an important predictor of pain and increased analgesic use. Pain catastrophizing scales (PCS), which include three subscales – rumination, magnification and helplessness – have been developed. A good correlation between PCS scores and pain perception has been demonstrated in a variety of chronic and acute pain states. As patient age increases, PCS scores decrease.

The meaning that a person attaches to pain can also influence their perception of pain intensity and the ability to tolerate pain. For example, perceived pain may be different if an operation for cancer is curative compared with one that is palliative only.

Anxiety and depression also seem to be important psychological variables affecting patient-controlled analgesia (PCA) use. Patients with preoperative anxiety or depression may have higher postoperative pain intensities and PCA analgesic consumption, as well as making more 'unsuccessful' PCA demands (i.e. during the 'lockout' interval).

Of course, under-treated pain can also lead to, or increase, patient anxiety, fear, sleeplessness and fatigue. Aggressive and belligerent behavior may be a sign of that anxiety and distress.

Locus of control testing may show how patients will respond and adapt to surgical pain. Those with an 'internal' locus of control believe that through their own behavior they can exert control over their health. A perception of lack of control in this group increases anxiety. Those with an 'external' locus of control believe that what they do will have little or no influence on the outcome of their health, and that their health is in the hands of fate, chance or other people. This latter group may be very dependent on the ward staff, and some may find the responsibility for control stressful.

Key points

Evidence level

III There is good correlation between the visual analogue and numerical rating scales

III Regular assessment of pain leads to improved acute pain management

IV Preoperative anxiety, catastrophizing, neuroticism and depression are associated with higher postoperative pain intensity

Clinical practice points

Self-reporting of pain should be used whenever appropriate, as pain is by definition a subjective experience

Scoring should incorporate different components of pain. In the postoperative patient this should include static (rest) and dynamic (e.g. pain on sitting, coughing) pain

Uncontrolled or unexpected pain requires a reassessment of the diagnosis and consideration of alternative causes for the pain (e.g. new surgical/medical diagnosis, neuropathic pain)

Reproduced with permission from Acute Pain Management: Scientific Evidence ANZCA and FPM (2005)

Assessment of adverse effects

In order to individualize treatment and maximize patient safety, there must be ongoing assessment of any adverse effects that might be related to pain management regimens.

The adverse effects and complications that can result from the treatment of acute pain will vary according to the drugs and techniques used, and are discussed in more detail in the chapters that follow. However, there are a number of parameters that should be monitored routinely in the acute pain setting if risk to patients is to be minimized. These include signs of excessive opioid doses, regardless of route of administration, and early signs of complications related to regional analgesia, particularly epidural analgesia (Box 3.3).

Respiratory depression

Respiratory depression is caused by direct action of the opioids on the respiratory center in the brain stem. It is a relatively uncommon (though

Box 3.3

Monitoring for adverse effects

Adverse effect	Comments
Respiratory depression (opioid related)	The best early clinical sign of opioid-related respiratory depression is increasing sedation
Oxygen saturation	In the non-sedated patient, decreases in blood oxygen saturation levels are most often due to causes other than opioids (e.g. pre-existing lung disease, obesity, postoperative changes in lung function and severe pain)
Hypotension	Hypotension associated with the use of opioid analgesics is often indicative of the presence of hypovolemia
	Hypotension associated with the use of epidural analgesia can be minimized if appropriate dose regimens are used (see Chapter 9)
	If appropriate dose regimens are used for epidural analgesia, hypotension in the acute pain setting often indicates the presence of hypovolemia

(Continued)

Box 3.3—cont'd

Monitoring for adverse effects

Adverse effect	Comments
Decreased motor and/or sensory function	Motor and sensory function should be assessed on a regular basis during any continuous regional analgesia, especially epidural analgesia
	Changes in motor and/or sensory function associated with epidural analgesia may be the first signs of an epidural hematoma or abscess
	Motor and sensory function should also be assessed for a period after removal of an epidural catheter
	Assessment of motor function should include asking the patient to flex their hip, i.e. unless the limb is injured, to draw their knee up to their chest. Assessment of movement at the ankle and toes only is not sufficient
Back pain	Increasing back pain may be the first sign of an epidural abscess following epidural or intrathecal analgesia
Urine output	In the acute pain setting a low urine output will often indicate concurrent hypovolemia
	NSAIDs and COX-2 selective inhibitors (see Chapter 6) should not be given until hypovolemia has been treated and urine output is satisfactory

much feared) complication of opioid administration. However, if doses are properly titrated, the risk is very small.

Although opioids have been used to treat acute pain for hundreds of years, there remains significant confusion about the best method of monitoring for respiratory depression. Measurement of arterial $P\text{CO}_2$ levels is the most accurate, but not possible in most patients, particularly on a regular basis. Therefore, reliance must be placed on clinical measures such as respiratory rate, oxygen saturation and increasing sedation.

Sedation score vs respiratory rate

Although still commonly used, a decrease in respiratory rate is known to be a late and unreliable sign of opioid-induced respiratory depression. A normal rate may coexist with marked respiratory depression, as inadequate ventilation can result from other opioid effects on the respiratory system (upper airway obstruction, a reduction in tidal volume or irregularities in respiratory rhythm; see Chapter 4). Hypoxemic episodes in the absence of a low respiratory rate have been shown to be common in patients given opioids.

As respiratory depression is almost always preceded by sedation, the best early clinical indicator of respiratory depression is increasing sedation, which can be monitored using a simple sedation score (Box 3.4). When the patient is asleep an assessment can usually be made without waking them fully (e.g. the patient turns when the pulse or blood pressure is taken).

In general, a respiratory rate of <8 breaths per minute is often considered to indicate respiratory depression. However, some patients may have rates as low as this or even lower, particularly when asleep, in the absence of respiratory depression. In some centers, respiratory rates of <8 per minute are tolerated as long as the patient is not sedated. As

---

Box 3.4

Commonly used indicators of respiratory depression

Sedation score	0	wide awake
	1	easy to rouse[*]
	2	constantly drowsy, easy to rouse but unable to stay awake (e.g. falls asleep during conversation); *early* respiratory depression
	3	severe; somnolent, difficult to rouse; *severe* respiratory depression
	[*]	some centers also add '1S', which indicates asleep but easy to rouse
Respiratory rate		Fewer than 8 breaths/min is often considered to be a sign of respiratory depression, but this is generally an unreliable indicator
		Respiratory depression can coexist with a normal respiratory rate
Oxygen saturation		May also be unreliable, especially if the patient is receiving supplemental oxygen

---

mentioned before, respiratory depression can coexist with a normal respiratory rate.

Regular assessment of level of sedation in any patient receiving opioids should be the '6th vital sign'.

Changes in Po_2, Pco_2 and oxygen saturation

Oxygen saturation (as measured by pulse oximetry) is used in many wards as an easy and non-invasive measure of blood oxygen levels. However, care must be taken in the interpretation of any readings. If the patient is receiving supplemental oxygen, the added oxygen may mask deterioration in respiratory function (i.e. 'normal' oxygen saturation levels may still be seen). Although low oxygen saturation levels in patients receiving oxygen indicate major abnormalities in respiratory function, normal oxygen saturation levels in patients receiving oxygen *do not* exclude abnormalities. In addition, unless continuous oxygen saturation monitoring is used, episodic hypoxemia may be missed.

For example, a healthy young patient before an operation given oxygen at 4 L/min may have an arterial Po_2 of 130–150 mmHg (17.3–20 kPa). The pulse oximeter may show an oxygen saturation of 99%. The same patient after a major abdominal operation and receiving the same amount of oxygen may have a Po_2 of only 100 mmHg (13.3 kPa), but the oximeter will show only a small decrease in saturation to 98%. Yet clearly there is an abnormality in lung function, leading to a lower than expected Po_2 for the inspired oxygen concentration. This would be even more obvious if a patient given oxygen at 10 L/min only had a Po_2 of 100 mmHg (13.3 kPa), far less than would be expected from this inspired oxygen concentration in normal lungs. The oxygen saturation would still be 98% despite obviously abnormal respiratory function.

The relationship between arterial Po_2 and oxygen saturation is not linear, due to the oxygen–hemoglobin dissociation curve (discussed in any physiology textbook). Some approximate values worth remembering are listed in Box 3.5.

If arterial blood gas analysis shows an increased arterial Pco_2, regardless of the Po_2 level, opioid-induced respiratory depression should be suspected.

Postoperative hypoxemia

Postoperative hypoxemia is reasonably common, especially after major surgery and in the elderly. It can be constant or episodic. In the non-sedated patient it is most often due to causes other than opioid medications.

Box 3.5

Relationship between arterial Po_2 and oxygen saturation

Arterial Po_2 (mmHg)	Arterial Po_2 (kPa)	Oxygen saturation (%)
100	13.3	98
90	12.0	97
80	10.7	95
70	9.3	93
60	8.0	90
40	5.3	75 (venous blood)
26	3.5	50

CONSTANT (BACKGROUND) HYPOXEMIA Reduced lung volumes, particularly vital capacity (VC) and functional residual capacity (FRC), are commonly seen after major surgery. The resultant airways closure, ventilation–perfusion abnormalities and atelectasis, which may be caused by a reduction in FRC, contribute to a constant hypoxemia that may last for a few days. Decreases in FRC peak at 24–48 hours postoperatively and usually resolve within a week. They persist, albeit to a lesser extent, even with complete pain relief. Risk factors for decreased FRC and postoperative hypoxemia include advanced age, upper abdominal and thoracic operations (and to a lesser extent other abdominal operations), obesity, pre-existing lung disease, smoking and severe pain. Patients after major orthopedic (joint replacement) surgery are also likely to be hypoxemic.

EPISODIC HYPOXEMIA With normal respiration, an increase in tone of the muscles of the upper airway precedes inspiration and helps maintain airway patency during the negative inspiratory pressures generated by chest and diaphragmatic actions. If the tonic or phasic activity of the upper airway muscles is reduced, as may occur during sleep or following the administration of opioids and/or benzodiazepines, closure of the upper airway on inspiration may result. This can manifest as snoring (partial upper airway obstruction) or complete upper airway obstruction (obstructive apnea).

Most obstructive apnea episodes take place during rapid eye movement (REM) sleep, which is also the phase in which most dreaming occurs. Patients who have obstructive sleep apnea (OSA) syndrome may have many obstructive episodes every hour. In the general population the prevalence of OSA is thought to be 5–10%. In the postoperative period, many more patients may fulfill the criteria for OSA syndrome.

Sleep patterns are often disturbed in the postoperative period or after non-surgical stress (e.g. severe injury, myocardial infarction). Typically, for the first night or two there is a reduction in total sleep time, elimination of REM sleep, a reduction in slow-wave (very deep non-REM) sleep and increased amounts of lighter, non-REM sleep. The disturbance in sleep patterns is greatest after major operations. Rebound REM sleep is typically seen during the second to fourth nights after surgery and is associated with more frequent episodes of airway obstruction than other sleep stages in the postoperative period. Vivid dreams and nightmares are more likely to occur during this increase in REM activity.

Marked reductions in the amount of slow wave sleep and REM sleep may also follow opioid administration, and any patient given opioids may have episodes of partial or complete airway obstruction when asleep (see Chapter 4).

Any episode of airway obstruction may lead to profound and rapid decreases in oxygen saturation, especially if patients already have a background hypoxemia. Unless continuous pulse oximetry is used, episodic hypoxemia is likely to be missed. Arterial P_{CO_2} levels may remain within normal limits.

COMPLICATIONS OF HYPOXEMIA Postoperative hypoxemia may lead to cardiac, cerebral and wound complications. Temporal relationships have been shown between episodic hypoxemia and myocardial ischemia, tachycardias and arrhythmias in the postoperative period. Hypoxemia may also lead to acute impairment of cognitive function (i.e. confusion or delirium), lowered resistance to infection, and impaired wound healing. As with rebound REM sleep and episodic hypoxemia, postoperative confusion and cardiac disturbances tend to be more common during the second to fourth nights after surgery.

POSTOPERATIVE SUPPLEMENTARY OXYGEN For the reasons outlined above it is often appropriate to administer oxygen in the postoperative period. Although there are no definite guidelines for dose and duration of therapy, routine oxygen administration for the first 2–4 days after surgery (and longer if indicated) has been suggested after major operations and in high-risk patients. Supplemental oxygen will not affect the number of episodes of intermittent hypoxemia but will reduce the degree of any background hypoxemia, providing an added safety margin should obstructive apnea develop. Nasal cannulae with oxygen flows of 2–4 L/min will be adequate for most patients and are more likely to stay in place than a face-mask.

Supplemental oxygen in the first 48 hours after major surgery is particularly beneficial in elderly and high-risk patients because of the link between postoperative delirium, tachycardia and myocardial ischemia.

It is possible that the benefits may also include reductions in other cardiovascular system and wound complications.

Pain antagonizes respiratory depression

Pain is an effective antagonist to opioid-induced respiratory depression. If a patient has received a large dose of opioid as treatment for pain and then, for example, a local anesthetic block is given to manage that pain, the onset of the block may be followed by respiratory depression. A similar result may follow if the cause of the pain is removed. For example, opioids self-administered by a patient using PCA for abdominal pain due to urinary retention may cause respiratory depression when a urinary catheter is inserted and the cause of the pain removed.

Key points

Evidence level

II Supplemental oxygen in the postoperative period improves oxygen saturation and reduces tachycardia and myocardial ischemia

IV Regular assessment of a patient's level of sedation is a more reliable clinical indicator of early opioid-induced respiratory depression than a decrease in respiratory rate

Reproduced with permission from Acute Pain Management: Scientific Evidence ANZCA and FPM (2005)

Motor and sensory function, back pain

The risks of epidural analgesia include the development of an epidural hematoma or abscess. This can result in nerve root and spinal cord compression and permanent neurological damage, including paraplegia (see Chapter 9). If a patient has an epidural catheter in situ, motor and sensory function should be monitored on a regular basis. Any reduction in function will usually be due to the local anesthetic in the epidural infusion. However, the presence of an epidural hematoma or abscess should always be excluded. This can be done by stopping the infusion for a time and checking that any deficit resolves. Motor and sensory function should also be checked for a period after removal of an epidural catheter.

Increasing back pain may be the first sign of an epidural abscess.

Other parameters

Other parameters requiring assessment in the acute pain setting include blood pressure, heart rate and urine output.

If a patient becomes hypotensive after receiving an opioid, regardless of route of delivery, the reason is usually that they are hypovolemic. Hypotension following epidural analgesia is often said to be more common, but if appropriate dose regimens are used (see Chapter 9), the incidence can be very low. Once again, hypotension often indicates an underlying hypovolemia. Bradycardia associated with epidural analgesia could indicate that the level of the block is at T1–T4, that is, at the level of the sympathetic nerves supplying the heart.

Urine output is also an important monitoring parameter. Not only might it be a sign of hypovolemia, but it should indicate caution with the administration of NSAIDs and COX-2 selective inhibitors (see Chapter 6). It is preferable to withhold these drugs until the hypovolemia is treated and urine output satisfactory.

References and further reading

Australian and New Zealand College of Anaesthetists, Faculty of Pain Medicine. Acute Pain Management: Scientific Evidence, 2nd edn. Melbourne: Australian and New Zealand College of Anaesthetists, 2005. Also available online at: *http://www.anzca.edu.au/publications/acutepain.htm* and *http://www7.health.gov.au/nhmrc/publications/synopses/cp104syn.htm*

Breivik EK, Bjornsson GA, Skovlund E. (2000) A comparison of pain rating scales by sampling from clinical trial data. Clinical Journal of Pain 16: 22–8.

Bouhassira D, Attal N, Alchaar H et al. (2005) Comparison of pain syndromes associated with nervous or somatic lesions and development of a new neuropathic pain diagnostic questionnaire (DN4). Pain 114: 29–36.

Cashman JN, Dolin SJ. (2004) Respiratory and haemodynamic effects of acute postoperative pain management: evidence from published data. British Journal of Anaesthesia 93: 212–23.

Catley DM, Thornton C, Jordan C et al. (1985) Pronounced, episodic oxygen desaturation in the postoperative period: its association with ventilatory pattern and analgesic regimen. Anesthesiology 63: 20–8.

Dawson R, Spross JA, Jablonski ES et al. (2003) Probing the paradox of patients' satisfaction with inadequate pain management. Journal of Pain and Symptom Management 23: 211–20.

DeLoach LJ, Higgins MS, Caplan AB et al. (1998) The visual analog scale in the immediate postoperative period: intrasubject variability and correlation with a numeric scale. Anesthesia and Analgesia 86: 102–6.

Dolin SJ, Cashman JN. (2005) Tolerability of acute postoperative pain management: nausea, vomiting, sedation, pruritus and urinary retention. British Journal of Anaesthesia 95: 589–91.

Granot M, Ferber SG. (2005) The roles of pain catastrophizing and anxiety in the prediction of postoperative pain intensity. Clinical Journal of Pain 21: 439–45.

Hobbs GJ, Hodgkinson V. (2003) Assessment, measurement, history and examination. In: Rowbotham DJ, Macintyre PE, eds. Clinical pain management: acute pain. London: Arnold.

JCAHO, NPC. (2001) Pain: current understanding of assessment, management and treatments. Joint Commission on Accreditation of Healthcare Organizations and the National Pharmaceutical Council, Inc. December 2001 (*http://www.jcaho.org/news+room/health+care+issues/pm+monographs.htm*)

Jensen MP, Mendoza T, Hanna DB et al. (2004) The analgesic effects that underlie patient satisfaction with treatment. Pain 110: 480–7.

Jones JG, Sapsford DJ, Wheatley RG. (1990) Postoperative hypoxia: mechanisms and time course. Anaesthesia 45: 566–73.

Kehlet H, Jensen TS, Woolf CJ. (2006) Persistent postsurgical pain: risk factors and prevention. Lancet 367: 1618–25.

Lynch M. (2001) Pain: the fifth vital sign. Comprehensive assessment leads to proper treatment. Advance for Nurse Practitioners 9: 28–36.

Mamie C, Morabia A, Bernstein M et al. (2000) Treatment efficacy is not an index of pain intensity. Canadian Journal of Anaesthesia 47: 1166–70.

Merskey H. (1979) Pain terms: a list with definitions and notes on usage. Recommended by the Subcommittee on Taxonomy. Pain 6: 249–52.

Morrison RS, Magaziner J, Gilbert M et al. (2003) Relationship between pain and opioid analgesics on the development of delirium following hip fracture. Journals of Gerontology. Series A, Biological Sciences and Medical Sciences 58: 76–81.

Olzap G, Sarioglu R, Tuncel G et al. (2003) Preoperative emotional states in patients with breast cancer and postoperative pain. Acta Anaesthiologica Scandinavica 47: 26–9.

Rosenberg J, Pedersen MH, Gebuhr P et al. (1992) Effect of oxygen therapy on late postoperative episodic and constant hypoxaemia. British Journal of Anaesthesia 68: 18–22.

Shapiro A, Zohar E, Zaslansky R et al. (2005) The frequency and timing of respiratory depression in 1524 postoperative patients treated with systemic or neuraxial morphine. Journal of Clinical Anesthesia 17: 537–42.

Stausholm K, Kehlet H, Rosenberg J. (1995) Oxygen therapy reduces postoperative tachycardia. Anaesthesia 50: 737–9.

Vila H, Smith RA, Augustyniak MJ et al. (2005) The efficacy and safety of pain management before and after implementation of hospital-wide pain treatment standards: is patient safety compromised by treatment based solely on numerical pain ratings? Anesthesia and Analgesia 101: 474–80.

4 Pharmacology of opioids

Opium and its preparations have been used to treat pain for over 2000 years. The psychological effects of opium were known to the ancient Sumerians for hundreds of years before that, and mention is made of its analgesic effect in Egyptian mythology. However, the first accepted reference to its use for the treatment of pain is found in the writings of Theophrastus in the third century BC.

Opium contains more than 25 different alkaloids, only two of which have any analgesic action: morphine (10% by weight of opium) and codeine (0.5% by weight). In 1806, Sertürner isolated the alkaloid of opium later called morphine (after Morpheus, the Greek god of dreams and son of Hypnos, god of sleep). Codeine was isolated in 1832. The introduction of the glass syringe and hollow needle in 1853 enabled the parenteral injection of morphine, facilitating its use, but also its abuse.

Morphine is still obtained from the opium poppy, *Papaver somniferum*, as its synthesis is expensive. Traditionally, opium is obtained by incising the unripe seed capsule of the poppy. However, this method of collection is very labor intensive and a more modern method of production harvests the dried poppy and extracts morphine, codeine and thebaine from the poppy straw.

Morphine remains the standard against which all new analgesics are compared. Although newer opioids may have different properties, particularly with regard to their pharmacokinetics, none is clinically superior in relieving pain. Therefore, many recent improvements in acute pain management have resulted from the better use of well-established opioids, rather than the use of newer drugs.

Drugs derived from the alkaloids of opium are called *opiates*. All drugs that have morphine-like actions, naturally occurring or synthetic, are called *opioids*. The term *narcotic*, derived from the Greek word for stupor, is also often used. However, this is probably best confined to a legal context, where it refers to a wide variety of drugs of addiction.

Tramadol is included in this chapter. Although it is strictly not a conventional opioid – it is better called an atypical centrally acting analgesic – part of its analgesic effect is mediated via opioid receptors. It is often used instead of conventional opioids.

Mechanisms of action

Until the mid-1970s very little was known about the mechanism of action of opioid drugs. Since then, not only have receptor sites for these drugs been identified, but it was also discovered that the body is capable of producing its own endogenous ligands for these receptors (i.e. endogenous opioids).

Endogenous opioids

Endogenous opioids identified so far are *endorphins, enkephalins, endomorphins* and *dynorphins*. They are found in the brain, spinal cord, gastrointestinal tract and plasma, and are released in response to stimuli such as pain or stress.

Opioid receptors

Opioid drugs produce their effect by acting as agonists at opioid receptors, which are found in the brain, spinal cord, and sites outside the central nervous system, including the urinary and gastrointestinal tracts, lung and peripheral nerve endings. There are three principal types of opioid receptor, mu (μ), delta (δ) and kappa (κ). The corresponding endogenous ligands (agonists) are β-endorphins, enkephalins and dynorphins, respectively. A sigma (σ) receptor was initially proposed and thought to mediate the dysphoric and psychotomimetic (hallucinations and delirium) effects of agonist–antagonist opioids. However, these effects are probably the result of κ receptor activity. The current suggested nomenclature and the effects of activation of the different receptors are summarized in Box 4.1.

The pharmacological effects of a given opioid are the result of its receptor specificity, receptor affinity and intrinsic activity at the various receptors. Whereas receptor affinity determines the amount of opioid needed to occupy a given percentage of receptors, it is the intrinsic activity of the opioid that determines its analgesic efficacy.

According to their intrinsic activity at the opioid receptors, opioid drugs are classed as:

- *agonists:* drugs that bind to and stimulate opioid receptors and are capable of producing a maximal response from the receptor (intrinsic activity 1);
- *antagonists:* drugs that bind to but do not stimulate opioid receptors and may reverse the effect of opioid agonists (intrinsic activity 0);

Box 4.1

Opioid receptor classification: current proposed terminology (IUPHAR Subcommittee)

Proposed nomenclature	Previous nomenclature	Endogenous ligands	Effects
μ, mu, or MOP1	OP3	β-endorphins, enkephalins, endomorphin-1, endomorphin-2	Analgesia, respiratory depression, euphoria, bradycardia, pruritus, miosis, nausea and vomiting, inhibition of gut motility, physical dependence
δ, delta, or DOP1	OP1	Enkephalins, β-endorphins	Analgesia
κ, kappa or KOP1	OP2	Dynorphin A, dynorphin B, α-neoendorphin	Analgesia, sedation, psychotomimetic effects, dysphoria, diuresis
NOP	OP4: ORL-1	Nociceptin, orphanine FQ	Not opioid-like

- *partial agonists:* drugs that stimulate opioid receptors but have a ceiling effect, i.e. produce a submaximal response compared with an agonist (intrinsic activity > 0 and < 1);
- *agonist–antagonists:* drugs that are agonists at one opioid receptor type and antagonists at another.

Placebo response

It is appropriate to discuss the issue of placebo response under the heading Mechanisms of Action, as a major component of the analgesic placebo response is mediated via the endogenous opioid system. It is well known that some patients will obtain pain relief from non-analgesic medications or interventions, or a greater than expected degree of relief from an analgesic drug or technique. This is known as the placebo analgesic response and it results, at least in part, from the release of endogenous opioids. This has been confirmed by observations that pain relief obtained from non-analgesic treatment is, at least to a significant degree, reversible by the administration of an opioid antagonist such as naloxone.

Effects of opioids

Analgesia

The major desirable effect of opioids is analgesia, which is mediated mainly via the μ receptor, although δ receptor effects can also contribute to pain relief. All full μ agonists are capable of producing the same degree of pain relief. Therefore, they can theoretically be made equianalgesic if adjustments are made for dose and route of administration (Box 4.2). However, it must be noted that standard equianalgesic dose tables present average data based on single-dose studies of the drugs in opioid-naive patients. They cannot account for interindividual differences in absorption, metabolism, and in some circumstances efficacy. Even more problematic is the use of such tables in patients on long-term opioid therapy, where factors such as incomplete cross-tolerance between opioids (see Chapter 14) and marked interpatient variability in the half-lives of the drugs or their active metabolites will have a significant effect on the total daily doses that may be required.

If a change is made from one opioid to another, particularly if high doses or long-term use have been necessary, it is suggested that the alternative be started at a lower than equianalgesic dose in the first instance. This increases the safety of the changeover; subsequent doses can then be titrated to effect.

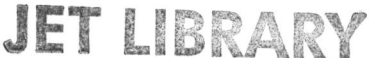

Box 4.2

Equianalgesic doses and half-lives of some commonly used opioids

Opioid	IM/IV (mg)	Oral (mg)	T$_{1/2}$ (h)
Morphine	10	30	2–3
Pethidine (meperidine)	100	400	3–4
Oxycodone	10	20	2–3
Codeine	130	200	2–4
Fentanyl	0.15–0.2	–	3–5
Alfentanil	0.75–1.5	–	1–2
Sufentanil	0.02	–	2–3
Diamorphine	5	60	0.5*
Methadone	10	10–15	15–40
Hydromorphone	1.5	7.5	3–4
Tramadol†	100	100	5–7
Buprenorphine	0.4	0.8 (S/L)‡	3–5
Pentazocine	60	150	3–5
Nalbuphine	10–20	–	2–4
Butorphanol	2	–	2–3

*Rapidly hydrolyzed to morphine.
† Only part of its analgesic action results from action on μ opioid receptors (see text).
‡ S/L, Sublingual.

NOTES:

- Table compiled from values obtained from listed references. Published reports vary in the suggested doses considered to be equianalgesic to morphine. Therefore, titration to clinical response in each patient is necessary.

- Suggested doses are the results of single dose studies only. Therefore, use of the data to calculate total daily dose requirements may not be appropriate.

- There may be incomplete cross-tolerance between these drugs. In patients who have been receiving one opioid for a prolonged period, it is usually necessary to use a dose lower than the expected equianalgesic dose when changing to another opioid, and to titrate to effect.

If a change is made from a parenteral route (intramuscular (IM), subcutaneous (SC) or intravenous (IV)) to the oral route of administration, the bioavailability of the opioid has to be considered. In general, larger doses will be needed orally because of the 'first-pass' effect: a proportion of an orally administered drug is metabolized by the liver and gut wall after absorption from the gastrointestinal tract. This effect diminishes the amount of unchanged drug that reaches the systemic circulation and hence the analgesic effect.

For all the above reasons, the conversions listed in Box 4.2 should be used as guidelines only. The list is limited to opioids in common use and not all will be available in every country. Furthermore, formulations, generic names and trade names may vary.

Most opioids have a similar spectrum of adverse effects that are linked mainly to µ receptor activation (Box 4.3). Clinical trials in acute pain management have shown that opioids administered in equianalgesic doses to large population groups have a similar incidence and degree of adverse effects. However, there may be individual differences in patient response, and some patients may experience more side effects with one particular drug. In these instances, opioid rotation, i.e. a change to another opioid, is appropriate.

Box 4.3

Possible side effects of opioids

Respiratory system	Respiratory depression, cough suppression, bronchoconstriction
Central nervous system	Sedation, euphoria (sometimes dysphoria), nausea and vomiting, miosis, muscle rigidity, myoclonus, seizures
Cardiovascular system	Vasodilatation, bradycardia, myocardial depression
Genitourinary system	Urinary retention
Gastrointestinal system	Delayed gastric emptying, constipation, spasm of the sphincter of Oddi
Pruritus	Possibly more common with morphine
Allergy	A 'true' allergy is uncommon

Effects on the respiratory system

Opioids cause a dose-dependent depression of all phases of respiratory activity. Therefore they affect the respiratory system in a number of ways and can lead to:

- a decrease in respiratory rate
- a decrease in tidal volume
- irregularities in respiratory rhythm, which may lead to periods of hypoventilation and central apnea, particularly when the patient is asleep
- intermittent partial or complete upper airway obstruction (obstructive apnea) when the patient is asleep.

Excessive doses of opioid may result in a progressive clinical respiratory depression; in doses that are not excessive, the last two effects in particular may lead to episodes of intermittent hypoxemia. Opioid-naive patients, patients at the extremes of age and those with pre-existing respiratory disease are at an increased risk of respiratory depression. Tolerance to respiratory depression develops rapidly.

It has been postulated that the respiratory centre also receives nociceptive input, so that pain acts as a physiological antagonist to respiratory depression. Therefore, if opioid doses are carefully titrated according to the pain the patient is experiencing, the risk of respiratory depression is very small. For details on the clinical relevance and the appropriate monitoring of respiratory depression related to opioid administration, see Chapter 3.

Opioids also directly inhibit the cough centre in the medulla and may be used for the treatment of cough. Although cough suppression might theoretically be a disadvantage in the postoperative period, this consideration should not limit the use of opioids in this setting.

Nausea and vomiting

Nausea and vomiting are very common adverse effects of opioids and are the most disturbing to patients. They occur as a result of activity in the vomiting center located in the brain stem. This center may be activated by stimuli from the chemoreceptor trigger zone (CTZ), upper gastrointestinal (GI) tract and pharynx, vestibular (motion) apparatus, and higher cortical areas (e.g. by olfactory, visual or emotional stimuli). The CTZ is outside the blood–brain barrier and is therefore exposed to any chemicals in the bloodstream. Opioids cause nausea and vomiting by stimulating opioid receptors in the CTZ and the GI tract; these effects are enhanced by vestibular stimulation. Opioids can also increase vestibular sensitivity, so that even slight movement, such as turning the head or moving in bed, may be enough to trigger nausea and vomiting in some patients.

Although the side-effect profiles of equianalgesic doses of opioids are similar, individual patients may report more postoperative nausea and vomiting (PONV) with one particular opioid. In this situation changing to another opioid (e.g. from morphine to fentanyl) is worth considering, especially when other measures, such as appropriate administration of antiemetics or a reduction in dose, have failed. It must be remembered that opioids are only one of many factors that can influence the incidence of PONV. Other factors include patient age, gender, phase of menstrual cycle, anxiety, a full stomach, type and duration of surgery, history of motion sickness or previous PONV, anesthetic drugs, and movement of the patient. Even unrelieved pain can be a cause of PONV. Patients should not be denied opioids in an attempt to treat or prevent PONV.

The incidence of PONV is still significant. It remains of major concern to patients and can significantly delay postoperative recovery, yet changes in attitudes concerning its treatment have lagged far behind those regarding pain management. Although there may be no benefit in giving *all* patients prophylactic antiemetics (in terms of either efficacy or cost), antiemetic therapy should be more aggressive in patients with established PONV.

There are a number of antiemetic drugs available and, like various classes of analgesic drug, they may differ with regard to site of action. Therefore, as with analgesic drugs, the use of a combination of antiemetic drugs that work at different receptor sites may be useful when a single drug has failed. Combinations of drugs with similar sites of action will increase the risk of side effects.

An alternative approach to 'PRN' administration (*pro re nata*, meaning 'according to circumstances' or 'as the situation requires') of antiemetics has been to add the drug (most commonly droperidol) to the opioid used in patient-controlled analgesia (PCA). However, large interpatient variations in postoperative opioid requirements mean that patients are likely to receive widely varying doses of the antiemetic. This could lead to inadequate therapy in some patients and an increased risk of side effects in others. In addition, the practice means that a significant proportion of patients will receive a drug they do not need. This has implications for cost as well as the potential for unnecessary side effects.

Despite the large number of antiemetic drugs available, PONV remains frustratingly difficult to treat in many patients. The 'perfect' antiemetic agent has yet to be found, and in some patients it is only 'tincture of time' that brings any relief.

Antiemetics

There are a number of different classes of antiemetic that act at the different receptor sites involved in the emetic response: dopamine, serotonin (5-hydroxytryptamine or $5HT_3$), acetylcholine (muscarinic type) and histamine, as well as corticosteroids. Failure of one class of drug should lead to the use of a drug from another class, droperidol, $5HT_3$ antagonists and dexamethasone being the most effective. Combinations of drugs from different classes can be helpful in otherwise intractable situations.

Antidopaminergic agents

Several different types of antiemetic drug have antidopaminergic actions, including butyrophenones (e.g. droperidol, haloperidol), phenothiazines (e.g. prochlorperazine) and the gastrointestinal prokinetic drug metoclopramide.

Droperidol is as effective as the $5HT_3$ inhibitors and dexamethasone for PONV. The adverse effects of butyrophenones are similar to those of phenothiazines and include extrapyramidal effects (ranging from restlessness and agitation to oculogyric crises) and the rare neuroleptic malignant syndrome. Some patients complain of marked apprehension. Lower doses may be as effective in the treatment of PONV as higher doses, but will have a lower incidence of side effects; a bolus dose of 0.5 mg droperidol is sufficient and has minimal adverse effects. Although there has been debate concerning the possibility that droperidol can cause prolongation of the QT interval and result in *torsades de pointes* arrhythmias in susceptible patients, a review of the reported cases could not establish a cause-and-effect relationship between low-dose droperidol (<1.25 mg) and such events.

Prochlorperazine has been used extensively for many years for the treatment of PONV. Potential side effects are those of any phenothiazine and include extrapyramidal reactions (which may occur after a single dose in some patients).

Metoclopramide acts centrally at dopamine receptors and peripherally to enhance gastric emptying. It also has some antagonistic effects at $5HT_3$ receptor sites. It is probably the most commonly used – albeit the least effective – antiemetic. In most studies it has consistently been shown to be less effective than $5HT_3$ inhibitors, droperidol and dexamethasone, and little more effective than placebo. Clinically, however, some patients appear to obtain relief (in some of these the nausea may have been a transient phenomenon only). The most important side effects associated with its use are extrapyramidal reactions, which can also occur after a single dose in some patients.

Antiserotinergic agents

These drugs (e.g. ondansetron, tropisetron and granisetron) are antagonists at the $5HT_3$ receptors. To date, they are the most effective antiemetics in nausea and vomiting induced by cytotoxic agents and among the most effective in PONV. Lack of extrapyramidal side effects and a longer duration of action are advantages, but cost can be a disadvantage. Because of pharmacodynamic and pharmacokinetic interactions, the co-administration of tramadol and ondansetron is not recommended; this may not be true for the more receptor-specific granisetron.

Anticholinergic agents

Scopolamine (hyoscine) has also been used to treat nausea and vomiting. It is available as a transdermal patch and is particularly effective for movement-induced nausea and vomiting; it may be associated with significant anticholinergic side effects, such as sedation, dry mouth, visual disturbances and confusion, and is not widely used in PONV.

Antihistamines

Antihistamines such as cyclizine, diphenhydramine, hydroxyzine and promethazine are commonly used as antiemetics and may be particularly effective for movement-induced PONV. Sedation may be a problem.

Steroids

Corticosteroids may also be very effective. Dexamethasone is now commonly used for the treatment of PONV, although usually as a single dose only.

Other effects on the central nervous system

Opioids cause constriction of the pupils (miosis); this is not necessarily an indication of an excessive dose. Although a mild euphoria may be associated with opioid administration, dysphoria occurs more often in the pain treatment setting.

Sedation and confusion

Mild sedation and cognitive impairment are common adverse effects of opioid therapy, especially just after the initiation of treatment, but tolerance develops rapidly. Untoward sedation suggests an excessive opioid dose and commonly precedes respiratory depression.

Postoperative confusion is often blamed on opioids, but opioids in therapeutic doses are usually not the cause – or at least not the sole cause. Other sources of confusion include sleep deprivation, hypoxia, withdrawal from alcohol or other drugs, sepsis, increasing age, endocrine and metabolic problems, and polypharmacy and drug interactions. Even unrelieved severe pain can result in confusion.

Initial treatment should aim at finding and treating any reversible cause. Hypoxemia is usually easily reversible and should be excluded in all cases. If pharmacological treatment of confusion is required, haloperidol is commonly the first drug of choice. It should be given in small, titrated doses. Benzodiazepines should be generally avoided because of the increased risk of respiratory depression if given in conjunction with opioids. However, they may be required in patients withdrawing from alcohol or at risk of withdrawing from benzodiazepines.

Rigidity, myoclonus and seizures

These adverse effects have occurred following rapid IV administration of large doses of opioids as well as with chronic oral therapy.

Muscle rigidity has only been reported after doses of opioids much larger than those routinely used in pain management.

One major cause of myoclonus and seizures is the accumulation of neurotoxic metabolites, particularly norpethidine, but also morphine-3-glucuronide – another important reason to avoid using pethidine, particularly in high doses or long term. Early reports suggested that tramadol could induce idiopathic seizures. However, later studies have shown that the risk of seizures following tramadol administration is no greater than with conventional opioids.

Overall, the risk of opioid-induced seizures seems to be dose related, although patients with pre-existing epilepsy or taking other seizure threshold-lowering drugs may be at increased risk. Clinical experience suggests that clonazepam is the agent of choice to terminate seizures induced by opioids.

Effects on the gastrointestinal and genitourinary systems

Opioids alter smooth muscle activity, leading to delayed gastric emptying, inhibition of bowel motility and constipation. This inhibition is both locally (an effect on opioid receptors in the bowel wall) and centrally mediated. Although some decrease in bowel motility is inevitable, it is usually not necessary or appropriate to withhold opioids to facilitate the return of bowel function after surgery. Adequate fluid intake and mobilization should be encouraged, and stool softeners and cathartics may be recommended (in the absence of contraindications) if opioids are to be given for more than a few days. Oral naloxone, or newer antagonists such as methylnaltrexone and, in particular, alvimopan (which has limited oral bioavailability and does not cross the blood–brain barrier) have been shown to reduce the effects of opioids on the bowel. Similarly, opioid agonists may also cause increases in biliary tract pressure and spasm of the sphincter of Oddi. This can be reversed by the administration of naloxone.

Urinary retention can occur owing to inhibition of the voiding reflex. This may also be reversed by naloxone, especially if it follows epidural or intrathecal opioid administration. It is not necessary for all patients receiving epidural or intrathecal opioid analgesia to be catheterized or to remain catheterized.

Effects on the cardiovascular system

Opioids can reduce vascular sympathetic tone, leading to hypotension. This is particularly likely in patients who have increased sympathetic tone, such as those with pain or poor cardiac function, some elderly patients, and patients who are hypovolemic. Opioids may also cause arterial and venous vasodilatation by a direct effect on vascular smooth muscle or through the release of histamine (notably morphine, diamorphine, pethidine and codeine). In clinical practice, and particularly in the postoperative period, a significant decrease in blood pressure following administration of an opioid in a supine patient often indicates that the patient is hypovolemic.

Opioids can also produce a vagally mediated bradycardia, but this is unlikely to be seen with the doses used in pain management. Pethidine may cause a slight tachycardia owing to its atropine-like effects. Postural (orthostatic) hypotension may occur when a supine patient given opioids sits or stands.

Pruritus

Some opioids, e.g. morphine, pethidine (meperidine) and codeine, cause the release of histamine from mast cells, resulting in local or generalized itching. This may be accompanied by flushing of the skin. If these opioids are given by IV injection, a localized urticaria may sometimes be seen at the site of injection or along the track of the vein into which the drug is being injected. This is due to local histamine release and does not usually indicate a true allergy to the opioid.

Although the exact mechanism of action is not known, pruritus due to opioids may also be centrally mediated, presumably a consequence of μ receptor activation at the dorsal horn level in the spinal cord. The itch is not associated with a rash and is not an allergic response to the drug. It is probably more common following morphine than pethidine or fentanyl, and is more likely following epidural or intrathecal administration of opioids. Itching is a common symptom and may not always be due to opioids. If it is opioid related, the patient will typically complain of itching over the face, neck and trunk. Itching confined mainly to the back is usually due to other causes.

Pruritus does not always require treatment. If the itching disturbs the patient, the safest treatment in the first instance is to change drugs (e.g. from morphine to fentanyl). Antihistamines (especially parenteral antihistamines) may add to the risk of sedation and respiratory depression. Pruritus may also respond to small, carefully titrated doses of IV naloxone. There is, however, a risk that naloxone will reverse the analgesia, although this is less likely if given following the administration of an epidural or intrathecal opioid. IV nalbuphine, in small doses, is also effective in some cases. The $5HT_3$ antagonist ondansetron has been used to treat pruritus in some patients, as has the anesthetic drug propofol.

Allergy

Patients and staff alike will often mistakenly report any adverse reaction to a drug as an allergy (e.g. nausea and vomiting following the administration of opioids). True allergic reactions to opioids are rare and are mediated by the immune system and result in signs and symptoms that are similar to other allergic reactions, including rash, urticaria, bronchoconstriction, angioneurotic edema and cardiovascular disturbances.

Predictors of opioid dose

Traditionally the dose of opioid prescribed for a patient has been based – if in fact it was based on anything – on the weight of the patient. In fact, there is no clinically significant correlation between weight and opioid requirement, and the best clinical predictor of opioid dose is the patient's age. Figure 4.1 shows the average IV PCA morphine requirements of

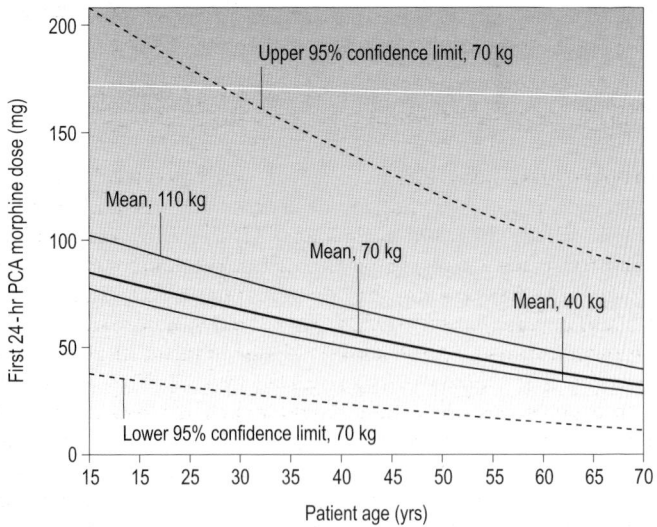

Figure 4.1 First 24-hour PCA morphine requirements and patient age. (Adapted with permission from Macintyre and Jarvis, 1996.)

1010 opioid-naive patients in the first 24 hours after major surgery. The total amount of morphine used in 24 hours decreases significantly as patient age increases. From Figure 4.1 it can be seen that the average first 24-hour morphine requirements were about 80 mg, 54 mg and 36 mg for patients aged 20 years, 45 years and 70 years, respectively. If a straight line is drawn through points representing 80 mg, 55 mg and 30 mg for these age groups (and the difference from the original points is well within the differences, owing to interpatient variation in each age group), it can be seen that after the age of 20 first 24-hour morphine requirements decrease by about 1 mg for each additional year of age, or:

average first 24-hour morphine requirements (mg) for patients over 20 years of age = 100 – (age in years)

Note the enormous variation (8–10-fold) in dose requirements in each age group. This means that although the initial dose of opioid should be based on the age of the patient, subsequent doses still need to be titrated to effect for each individual.

Although the weight of the patient has some effect on dose it is clinically insignificant compared with the overall interpatient variation.

There are a number of reasons why the dose of opioid required for pain relief should decrease with patient age. These include age-related changes in pharmacokinetics (how the individual handles the drug, e.g. distribution, metabolism and elimination) and pharmacodynamics (how the individual responds to the drug, e.g. perception of pain). However, it is the latter (i.e. pharmacodynamics) that are thought to play the largest part in the age-related decrease in opioid requirements.

Titration of opioid dose

For an opioid to be effective it must reach a certain blood level (this applies to systemically administered opioids and not to epidural and intrathecal opioids, which are discussed in Chapter 9). The effective range of blood concentrations varies widely between patients. The amount of opioid that each patient requires will also vary according to the severity of the pain stimulus. Thus titration is needed in order to individualize treatment.

The lowest concentration of opioid that will produce analgesia is known as the *minimum effective analgesic concentration* (MEAC). This varies widely between patients, but also within individual patients, depending on the severity of pain and possibly psychological factors. MEAC should therefore not be regarded as a static number, but more as a concept. Below the MEAC a patient will experience poor pain relief and above it there will be increasing analgesia, but also an increasing possibility of side effects. In reality, the boundaries are somewhat blurred and side effects may occur before good pain relief is obtained. The therapeutic range of blood levels (where analgesia is achieved without significant side effects) is often colloquially referred to as the 'analgesic corridor' (Figure 4.2). For each patient the aim of titration is to find and then maintain the effective blood level within this 'corridor'. A change in pain intensity may shift the corridor and require an increase or decrease in opioid dose.

To enable opioid analgesia to be titrated for each patient, appropriate doses and dose intervals need to be ordered. In addition, endpoints that indicate adequate or excessive doses need to be monitored repeatedly.

Dose interval

When an interval between intermittent doses of opioid is prescribed, the aim is primarily to allow the full effect of the previous dose to be seen before another dose may be given. It is also often used to give an indication of the expected duration of action of the drug, although choosing dosing intervals based on this parameter will not allow appropriate and effective titration.

The speed of onset of effect of an opioid will be influenced by its route of administration and its lipid solubility. The time taken for an opioid to reach a maximum blood concentration depends primarily on the route of administration. However, the time taken to then achieve maximum effect depends on the rate at which the drug crosses to the central nervous system and opioid receptors. Factors that determine the rate of this transfer include the lipid solubility of the drug (Box 4.4) and the concentration gradient. Of the opioids in common clinical use, morphine is the least

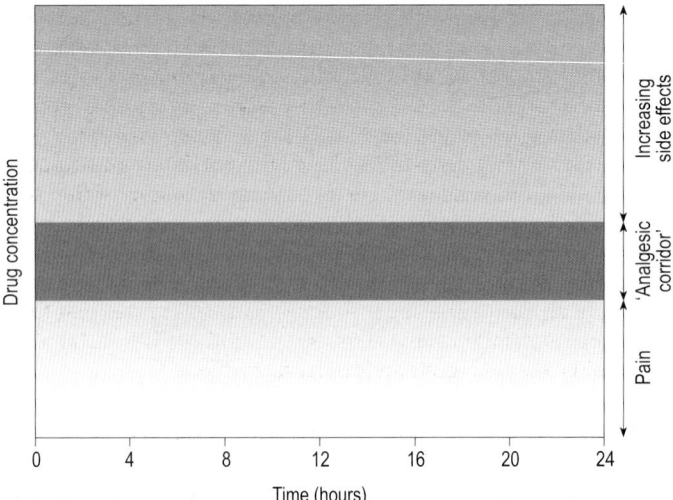

Figure 4.2 'Analgesic corridor'.

Box 4.4

Lipid solubilities of some of the commonly used opioids

Opioid	Lipid solubility[*]
Morphine	1
Pethidine (meperidine)	39
Fentanyl	813
Alfentanil	129
Sufentanil	1780
Diamorphine	280
Methadone	116
Hydromorphone	1.4

[*]Octanol/pH 7.4 buffer partition coefficient.
Values may vary according to different references.

lipid soluble and has the longest delay: it may take up to 15 minutes or more following an IV injection for its maximum effect to be seen. The full effect of IV fentanyl, on the other hand, may be seen within 5 minutes. Although less lipid soluble than fentanyl, the maximum effect of alfentanil may be seen within 1–2 minutes. This is because of the much greater proportion of alfentanil present in a non-ionized form. The time to peak effect needs to be taken into account when dose intervals are prescribed.

The duration of action of any given dose of opioid also depends on a number of factors, including the amount given, the route of administration, and the pharmacokinetic characteristics of the drug, such as absorption, rate of distribution to different tissues (including receptors), rate of dissociation from receptors, lipid solubility and elimination half-life. The elimination half-life alone does not determine duration of action. It is the time taken for the blood concentration of the drug to change by 50%, and gives an indication of the rate at which the body metabolizes and excretes the drug.

Drugs are metabolized to a form that is more easily excreted. In the case of opioids, the liver is the primary site of metabolism and the kidney the primary route of excretion of metabolites. The metabolites of some opioids have analgesic and/or adverse effects.

Monitoring of pain and sedation scores and other side effects

When titrating any drug, ongoing monitoring of endpoints that indicate 'how much is enough' and 'how much is too much' is necessary.

The best way to monitor the former is to use a pain score and functional assessment. The most serious consequence of excessive opioid dose is respiratory depression, and the best early indication of this is sedation. Nausea and vomiting or lightheadedness may also indicate a slightly excessive dose. For more detail on assessment and monitoring see Chapter 3.

The aim of pain treatment is to make the patient comfortable while keeping the sedation score below 2 (Box 4.5). If the patient does become sedated, subsequent doses should be reduced. If the patient is uncomfortable and not sedated, a larger dose may be required. Although many guidelines suggest that the respiratory rate should be maintained at above 8 breaths per minute, there may be occasions when a lower rate can be tolerated, provided the patient is not sedated.

Commonly used opioid agonists

Codeine

Codeine is a naturally occurring alkaloid like morphine. It is metabolized in the liver, where about 2–10% of the dose is converted to morphine. This accounts for all the analgesic effect of codeine, as the drug itself has a very low affinity for opioid receptors. It should therefore be regarded as an ineffective *prodrug* of morphine. Metabolism to morphine involves the enzyme CYP 2D6, which is an isoenzyme of the

---

Box 4.5

Basic requirements for opioid titration

For each route of opioid administration, safe and effective titration requires:

- Initial prescription of the appropriate age-related dose range
- Use of a dose interval (the interval where additional doses should not be given) appropriate to the route of administration
- Regular monitoring of pain and sedation scores
- Monitoring for the presence of other adverse effects
- Alteration of subsequent doses according to patient response (pain relief and adverse effects)

Aims for:

Patient comfort (not necessarily pain free), sedation score < 2 and respiratory rate <8 breaths/min (in most cases)

---

cytochrome P450 system; 8–10% of the Caucasian population are thought to lack this enzyme, and these patients will obtain no pain relief from codeine.

Codeine is usually given for the treatment of mild to moderate pain by intramuscular or oral routes. There are a number of oral formulations that combine codeine with non-opioid analgesics such as paracetamol (acetaminophen) or aspirin; these show increased analgesic efficacy, but also more opioid-related adverse effects.

Diamorphine (heroin)

Diamorphine does not bind to opioid receptors and has no analgesic activity. It is a *prodrug* and is rapidly hydrolyzed to 6-monoacetylmorphine (a potent analgesic) and then morphine. It has not been shown to have any clinical advantage over morphine when administered parenterally. Both diamorphine and 6-monoacetylmorphine are more lipid soluble than morphine; this is perceived as an advantage when administered via the epidural route. Diamorphine is available for medical use only in the UK.

Fentanyl and its analogs

Fentanyl is a highly lipid-soluble synthetic opioid that does not cause histamine release. It has a more rapid onset of action than morphine, and single doses have a short duration of action because of rapid tissue uptake from plasma. The metabolites of fentanyl are inactive, and therefore fentanyl is a good choice of opioid in patients with renal impairment.

For the treatment of acute pain fentanyl can be administered intravenously (for example by PCA), epidurally or intrathecally. Oral transmucosal ('lollipop') administration has been used in children and to treat breakthrough pain in cancer patients; true oral administration is not effective because of the very high first-pass effect. The high lipid solubility of fentanyl makes it suitable for transdermal administration (see Chapter 7).

Alfentanil and sufentanil are both highly lipid soluble. They have a more rapid onset and a shorter duration of action than fentanyl, despite the lower lipid solubility of alfentanil. This makes them very suitable for administration by IV infusion during anesthesia, but probably of limited use in the postoperative period. They have been used either alone or in combination with local anesthetics agents, for epidural analgesia. Both drugs are primarily eliminated by the liver.

A newer opioid, remifentanil, has very rapid onset. It also has an ultrashort duration of action owing to its metabolism by non-specific blood and tissue esterases. It is mainly used in clinical practice as an infusion during anesthesia. Depending on the type of surgery, postoperative pain may be significant unless postoperative analgesic strategies are introduced before the remifentanil infusion is stopped. In addition, there is some evidence that intraoperative use of high-dose remifentanil induces acute opioid tolerance and possibly hyperalgesia, resulting in increased postoperative pain intensity and opioid requirements.

Hydrocodone

Hydrocodone is available in the USA in combination formulations with non-opioid analgesics such as paracetamol, which limits the amount of the opioid that can be given. Its half-life is similar to that of codeine.

Hydromorphone

A semisynthetic opioid (a direct derivative of morphine), hydromorphone is available in oral, parenteral and suppository forms and can also be used for epidural analgesia. It has no active (analgesic) metabolites. However, the metabolite hydromorphone-3-glucuronide shows similar neurotoxic effects to M3G, and its excretion is dependent on renal function. Hydromorphone is around five times as potent as morphine.

Methadone

A synthetic opioid developed during World War II, methadone has a much longer half-life than other opioids and therefore a much longer duration of action. These properties make methadone more suitable for the management of chronic pain, or of a patient with an opioid substance abuse disorder, than for the treatment of acute pain.

Single doses of methadone may produce a quality and duration of analgesia similar to those of a single equianalgesic dose of morphine (see Box 4.2). However, the long half-life of methadone means that significant accumulation of drug can occur in an unpredictable fashion, and the large interindividual variability in total daily dose requirements makes methadone more difficult to use than other opioids. If a patient has been taking another opioid for some time and is changed to methadone, the dose should start at about 10% of the calculated equianalgesic dose for single administration and then be titrated to effect.

Methadone is thought to be an NMDA receptor antagonist (see Chapter 6) and have additional monaminergic effects. It may be of use in the treatment of neuropathic pain (see Chapter 12). It can be given by oral, IV, SC, IM and epidural routes.

Morphine

Morphine is the least lipid soluble of all opioids in common use. It is metabolized principally in the liver and less than 10% is excreted unchanged by the kidneys.

The main metabolites of morphine, morphine 6-glucuronide (M6G) and morphine 3-glucuronide (M3G), have longer half-lives than morphine and are excreted primarily via the kidney. Morphine 6-glucuronide is a more potent μ receptor agonist than morphine and may contribute significantly to its analgesic effect, particularly in patients on long-term morphine therapy. It may have a different spectrum of side effects from morphine, possibly owing to structural similarities to buprenorphine. In patients with reduced renal function the half-life of morphine is not significantly increased. However, there may be an apparent prolongation of its effect (and its adverse effects) owing to the accumulation of M6G.

Morphine 3-glucuronide has no analgesic activity and does not appear to compete for opioid receptor-binding sites. It may even antagonize the analgesic effects of morphine and M6G, although this is not yet clear. There is some evidence that M3G may influence the development of morphine tolerance, and that it might be responsible for some of the side effects seen with long-term high-dose morphine treatment, such as myoclonus, seizures, hyperalgesia and allodynia.

Morphine can be given by intramuscular, IV, SC, oral, transmucosal, rectal, epidural and intrathecal routes. Dose ranges and intervals will vary according to the route of administration.

Slow-release (also called controlled-release or sustained-release) preparations of oral morphine are available and often used in the treatment of chronic and cancer pain. They only need to be given one to two, sometimes three times a day. The slower onset (3–4 hours or longer) and prolonged duration of action of these formulations make fast titration of the drug impossible, so these preparations are usually unsuitable for the treatment of acute pain, at least in the initial stages.

Oxycodone

Oxycodone has been in clinical use since 1917; it is a thebaine derivative. Because it was first introduced into many countries in oral formulations combined with paracetamol (acetaminophen) or aspirin (similar to codeine), it was often considered suitable for the treatment of mild to moderate pain only. However, like all pure opioid agonists it has no ceiling effect for analgesia, is more potent than morphine, and in higher doses can be used for the treatment of severe pain.

The major metabolite of oxycodone is noroxycodone, which has only minimal analgesic activity and is renally excreted. Oxymorphone, another metabolite, possesses significant analgesic activity. However, it is present only in very low concentrations and contributes little to the pain-relieving effect of oxycodone. The formation of oxymorphone, but not noroxycodone, depends on the enzyme CYP 2D6 (see codeine above).

Oxycodone can be given by parenteral, oral and rectal routes. A slow-release formulation of oral oxycodone is available which has a fast-release component and therefore a quicker onset of action than currently available slow-release morphine preparations.

Pethidine (meperidine)

Pethidine was first synthesized just prior to World War II as a potential substitute for atropine. In addition to its analgesic effect, pethidine has some atropine-like actions that may lead to a dry mouth or slight tachycardia, and some local anaesthetic activity (this latter effect has allowed intrathecal pethidine to be used as the sole agent for spinal anesthesia). Myocardial depression can occur with larger doses. In patients taking monoamine oxidase inhibitors, hyperpyrexia, convulsions, coma and hypertension or hypotension have been reported following the administration of pethidine. Pethidine is thought to have a weak affinity for the N-methyl-D-aspartate (NMDA) receptor (see Chapter 6).

Pethidine can be given by IM or IV injection or infusion (SC injections may be excessively painful) as well as by oral, rectal, transmucosal, epidural and intrathecal routes. As with morphine, the range of doses and dose durations required will vary according to the route of administration. Although there is a widespread belief that pethidine is superior to other opioids such as morphine for the treatment of renal or biliary colic, the evidence shows that all opioids are equally effective.

Pethidine has been used to treat shivering associated with volatile anesthetic agents, epidural and spinal anesthesia, and chemotherapy. The usual initial dose is 12–25 mg IV.

Pethidine is metabolized primarily in the liver and the metabolites are excreted by the kidney. Less than 10% of pethidine is excreted unchanged by the kidneys. One of the main metabolites is norpethidine (normeperidine), which has a long half-life of 15–20 hours. A build-up of this metabolite can lead to norpethidine neurotoxicity.

Norpethidine is a μ agonist and therefore an analgesic, but it also has other non-opioid effects. High blood levels can lead to signs of central nervous system (CNS) excitation, including anxiety, mood change,

Box 4.6

Norpethidine (normeperidine) toxicity

Effects of norpethidine	Analgesia (μ receptor mediated)
	CNS excitation (non-opioid effect)
Half-life ($T_{1/2}$)	15–20 hours
Signs and symptoms	Anxiety, agitation, mood change, tremors, twitching, myoclonic jerks, convulsions
Treatment	Discontinue pethidine
	Substitute an alternative opioid
	Symptomatic treatment of effects
	DO NOT administer naloxone
Dose limits (suggested)	1000 mg in first 24 hours
	600–700 mg/day thereafter These dose limits should be reduced in the elderly; the drug should be avoided in patients with renal impairment

tremors, twitching, myoclonic jerks and even frank convulsions (Box 4.6). Patients receiving large doses of pethidine or those with renal impairment are particularly at risk.

Signs of norpethidine toxicity can be seen within 24–36 hours in some healthy patients with normal renal function who have required doses of pethidine that are in the higher range for each age group. There is no specific treatment for norpethidine toxicity. Pethidine should be discontinued and another opioid substituted. Naloxone should not be given, as it will antagonize the sedative effect of pethidine but not the excitatory effects of norpethidine. It will therefore only exacerbate the problem.

As there is no specific treatment, it is important to watch for early signs and symptoms of toxicity and prevent excessive levels of norpethidine by limiting the amount of pethidine administered. It is difficult to predict exactly what dose of pethidine or what blood level of norpethidine is likely to cause norpethidine toxicity in any particular patient. However, it is suggested that young patients with normal renal function should not receive more than 1000 mg in the first 24 hours of treatment. Subsequent totals should probably not exceed 600–700 mg per 24 hours. These limits should be reduced for elderly patients, and the drug should be avoided in patients with renal impairment.

The best treatment is prevention and the avoidance of the use of pethidine for the treatment of pain, especially as it seems to show an increased risk of drug-seeking behaviors in patients exposed to it (partially due to its high lipophilicity).

Propoxyphene

Structurally similar to methadone, only the dextrorotatory (*R* isomer) form has any analgesic activity (dextropropoxyphene). Often administered in an oral formulation in combination with paracetamol (acetaminophen) or aspirin, these preparations may be no more effective than paracetamol or aspirin alone. Toxicity, with hallucinations, delusions and confusion, may occur with accumulation of the renally excreted active metabolite norpropoxyphene, particularly in the elderly or those with renal impairment. Cardiotoxicity has also been reported, with prolongation of the QT interval and the risk of *torsades de pointes*. In view of these significant disadvantages and risks, dextropropoxyphene is currently in the process of being removed from the UK market by the regulatory authorities.

The half-lives of dextropropoxyphene and nordextropropoxyphene are respectively 6–12 hours and more than 30 hours, and may be even longer in the elderly.

Tramadol

Tramadol is a centrally acting synthetic analgesic agent. It has some μ receptor activity, mediated through its main metabolite *O*-desmethyltramadol (M1), and also inhibits the reuptake of norepinephrine (noradrenaline) and serotonin (5-hydroxytryptamine, 5HT) at nerve terminals. These mechanisms account for about 40%, 40% and 20%, respectively, of its activity. The latter effect – inhibition of norepinephrine and serotonin reuptake – is similar to the mechanism of action of tricyclic antidepressants (TCAs) and explains the efficacy of tramadol in neuropathic pain (see Chapter 12). As the analgesic effect of tramadol is only partially mediated via opioid receptor effects, it is not suitable as a replacement for conventional opioids in patients who are opioid dependent.

The main advantages over equianalgesic doses of other conventional opioids are less sedation and respiratory depression and less constipation; the incidence of nausea and vomiting is similar. In addition, the abuse potential of tramadol is minimal and it is therefore not a controlled drug. A history of epilepsy may be a relative contraindication to its use as seizures have been reported, although the incidence is probably similar to that of other opioids.

Although the combination of tramadol with SSRIs or TCAs may theoretically increase the risk of serotonin syndrome, this complication is rarely seen in the doses commonly used clinically. Tramadol should not be given in combination with monoamine oxidase (MAO) inhibitors.

Tramadol is available in oral and parenteral forms. As bioavailability following oral administration is high, doses are similar for both oral and parenteral routes. Product information sheets limit the total daily dose to 600 mg, although much higher doses have been used successfully worldwide. There is no advantage in neuraxial administration of tramadol and this route should be avoided, as data on neurotoxicity are incomplete.

As noted above, the main active metabolite of tramadol is O-desmethyl-tramadol (M1). M1 is a μ receptor agonist and is more potent than tramadol itself, thereby contributing to its analgesic efficacy. The formation of M1 depends on the enzyme CYP 2D6; in poor metabolizers the analgesic effect of tramadol is reduced (see Codeine, above). The accumulation of M1 in renal failure has been described as the cause of respiratory depression with tramadol, as it is excreted by the kidney.

Partial agonists and agonist–antagonists

Partial agonists have an affinity for opioid receptors but not the intrinsic activity of full agonists. When given in doses that are equianalgesic to full agonists these drugs have the same side effects, but there is a ceiling effect for both analgesia and adverse effects. This limits their clinical usefulness.

Agonist–antagonist drugs derive their analgesic actions principally from the activation of one opioid receptor, while acting as antagonists at another.

These drugs are said to have a lower potential for abuse than other opioids, but this is of limited significance in patients with no previous history of substance abuse and in whom the risk of addiction to opioids used for the treatment of acute pain is minimal. The agonist–antagonist drugs can precipitate withdrawal signs and symptoms in opioid-dependent patients.

On the whole, partial agonist and agonist-antagonist opioid drugs are used far less commonly in clinical practice than the pure opioid agonist drugs.

Buprenorphine

Buprenorphine is derived from the opium alkaloid thebaine and is available in parenteral, sublingual and transdermal formulations. It is highly lipid soluble, hence its excellent absorption by the sublingual route. It has high affinity for and dissociates slowly from the μ receptor, therefore its potency is high and the duration of action may be prolonged. In addition, it is an antagonist at the κ receptor.

Buprenorphine is available as a transdermal preparation for the treatment of chronic and cancer pain. It is also increasingly used as an opioid substitute in the management of patients with an opioid substance abuse disorder (see Chapter 14).

Buprenorphine behaves very differently from full opioid agonists; the data available remain confusing and further research is necessary. In animals, it shows a bell-shaped dose–response curve for analgesia – that is, a ceiling effect has been demonstrated for analgesia, meaning that once a certain dose level is reached the administration of further doses will not result in better pain relief. In humans, no ceiling effect for analgesia has been observed over a dose range from 0.05 to 0.6 mg, but there is a ceiling for adverse effects, in particular respiratory depression and sedation. Possible explanations, among others, are a difference in opioid receptor density in different parts of the CNS, or effects on the NOP receptor.

In case of an overdose, buprenorphine can be reversed by naloxone; however, significantly higher doses than usual (in the range of 2–4 mg) and a subsequent continuous infusion may be required.

Pentazocine

Pentazocine was the first drug of this class to become established in clinical practice. It can be given orally or parenterally. The high incidence of dysphoria associated with the drug has limited its use.

Nalbuphine

Chemically related to naloxone, nalbuphine is available as a parenteral preparation. It may be effective in reversing some of the side effects of μ-agonist drugs, such as respiratory depression and pruritus. However, its clinical use is rather limited and many studies aiming to show a 'sequential' analgesic effect of this drug were disappointing.

Butorphanol

Butorphanol is available as parenteral and intranasal preparations.

Opioid antagonists

These drugs are antagonists at all receptor sites; the most commonly used is naloxone.

Naloxone

Naloxone is the opioid antagonist most commonly used to treat opioid overdose. Its half-life – about 60 minutes – is much shorter than that of the drugs listed above. As a result, if naloxone is required to antagonize the effects of most opioid agonists, repeated doses or an infusion may be needed. By titrating the dose of naloxone, it is possible to reverse opioid-related respiratory depression, excessive sedation, nausea and vomiting, and pruritus while still retaining reasonable analgesia. However, this balance may be more difficult to obtain when opioids are being administered by other than epidural or intrathecal routes.

For the treatment of respiratory depression and excessive sedation, 40–100 μg of naloxone should be given intravenously and repeated every few minutes as required. If no venous access is available, the drug can be given in larger doses (e.g. 400 μg) by SC or IM injection. Smaller doses may be more suitable if naloxone is used to reverse other side effects of opioids. If a patient is on chronic opioid therapy, it is especially important to titrate naloxone in order to avoid precipitating withdrawal signs and symptoms.

Although some cardiovascular stimulation (hypertension, tachycardia) or nausea and vomiting may be seen after naloxone administration, especially after rapid reversal of analgesia, serious side effects such as pulmonary edema and arrhythmias are rare.

Naloxone is poorly absorbed following oral administration, and can therefore be used orally for the treatment of opioid-induced constipation. It can also be added to oral opioid preparations to make them unsuitable for parenteral abuse (for example in some preparations of buprenorphine used in drug substitution programs for patients with an opioid substance abuse disorder).

Naltrexone

Unlike naloxone, naltrexone is effective when given orally. It has a half-life of 2–4 hours and its main metabolite is 6-naltrexol, a weaker μ antagonist but with a half-life of more than 8 hours. Naltrexone (either orally or in the form of a subcutaneous implant) has been used in the treatment of opioid addiction, where the effects of a 50 mg dose may last up to 24 hours (see Chapter 14). It has also been used in the treatment of alcoholism.

Alvimopan

Alvimopan is a μ receptor antagonist which was developed for the prevention and/or treatment of opioid-induced ileus and constipation. It shows very limited oral bioavailability and no penetration of the blood–brain barrier. Its main effect is on receptors in the gut wall, where it has a higher affinity than naloxone. It has an adverse effect profile similar to that of placebo, but accelerates the recovery of GI function after surgery and reduces opioid-induced bowel dysfunction in chronic pain patients.

Key points

Evidence level

I Dextropropoxyphene has low analgesic efficacy

I Tramadol is an effective treatment for neuropathic pain

I Droperidol, dexamethasone and ondansetron are equally effective in prophylaxis of postoperative nausea and vomiting

I Naloxone, naltrexone, nalbuphine and droperidol are effective treatments for opioid-induced pruritus

II In the management of acute pain, one opioid is not superior over others but some opioids are better in some patients

II The incidence of clinically meaningful adverse effects of opioids is dose-related

II Tramadol has a lower risk of respiratory depression and impairs gastrointestinal motor function less than other opioids at equianalgesic doses

II Pethidine is not superior to morphine in treatment of pain of renal or biliary colic

IV In adults, patient age rather than weight is a better predictor of opioid requirements, although there is a large interpatient variation

IV Impaired renal function and the oral route of administration result in higher levels of the morphine metabolites M3G and M6G

Clinical practice points

Assessment of sedation level is a more reliable way of detecting early opioid-induced respiratory depression than a decreased respiratory rate.

The use of pethidine should be discouraged in favor of other opioids.

References and further reading

Andersen G, Christrup L, Sjogren P. (2003) Relationships among morphine metabolism, pain and side effects during long–term treatment: an update. Journal of Pain and Symptom Management 25: 74–91.

Apfel CC, Korttila K, Abdalla M et al. (2004) A factorial trial of six interventions for the prevention of postoperative nausea and vomiting. New England Journal of Medicine 350: 2441–51.

Australian and New Zealand College of Anaesthetists, Faculty of Pain Medicine. Acute Pain Management: Scientific Evidence, 2nd edn. Melbourne: Australian and New Zealand College of Anaesthetists, 2005. Also available online at: *http://www.anzca.edu.au/publications/acutepain.htm* and *http://www7.health.gov.au/nhmrc/publications/synopses/cp104syn.htm*

Dahan A, Yassen A, Romberg R et al. (2006) Buprenorphine induces ceiling in respiratory depression but not in analgesia. British Journal of Anaesthesia 96: 627–32.

Gan TJ, Meyer T, Apfel C et al. (2003) Consensus guidelines for managing postoperative nausea and vomiting. Anesthesia and Analgesia 97: 62–71.

Inturrisi CE. (2002) Clinical pharmacology of opioids for pain. Clinical Journal of Pain 18: S3–13.

Johnson RE, Fudala PJ, Payne R. (2005) Buprenorphine: considerations for pain management. Journal of Pain and Symptom Management 29: 297–326.

Jones JG, Sapsford DJ, Wheatley RG. (1990) Postoperative hypoxia: mechanisms and time course. Anaesthesia 45: 566–73.

Kalso E. (2005) Oxycodone. Journal of Pain and Symptom Management 29: S47–56.

Kjellberg F, Tramer MR. (2001) Pharmacological control of opioid-induced pruritus: a quantitative systematic review of randomized trials. European Journal of Anaesthesiology 18: 346–57.

Latta K S, Ginsberg B, Barkin RL. (2002) Meperidine: a critical review. American Journal of Therapeutics 9: 53–68.

Leslie JB. (2005) Alvimopan for the management of postoperative ileus. Annals of Pharmacotherapy 39: 1502–10.

Macintyre PE, Jarvis DA. (1996) Age is the best predictor of postoperative morphine requirements. Pain 64: 357–64.

Mather LE, Woodhouse A. (1997) Pharmacokinetics of opioids in the context of patient controlled analgesia. Pain Reviews 4: 20–32.

Mercadante S, Arcuri E. (2004) Opioids and renal function. Journal of Pain 5: 2–19.

Murray A, Hagen NA. (2005) Hydromorphone. Journal of Pain and Symptom Management 29: S57–66.

Peng WH, Sandler AN. (1999) A review of the use of fentanyl analgesia in the management of acute pain in adults. Anesthesiology 90: 576–99.

Roberts DM, Meyer-Witting M. (2005) High-dose buprenorphine: perioperative precautions and management strategies. Anaesthesia and Intensive Care. 33: 17–25.

Rosenberg-Adamsen S, Kehlet, Dodds C et al. (1996) Postoperative sleep disturbances: mechanisms and clinical implications. British Journal of Anaesthesia 76: 552–9.

Scott LJ, Perry CM. (2000) Tramadol: a review of its use in perioperative pain. Drugs 60: 139–76.

Schug SA. (2003) Tramadol in acute pain. Acute Pain 5: 1–2.

Schug SA, Gandham N. (2006) Opioids: Clinical use. In: McMahon SB, Koltzenburg M, eds. Wall and Melzack's textbook of pain, 5th edn. Amsterdam: Elsevier.

Stone PA, Macintyre PE, Jarvis DA. (1993) Norpethidine toxicity and patient-controlled analgesia. British Journal of Anaesthesia 71: 738–40.

Tramèr M. (2001) A rational approach to the control of postoperative nausea and vomiting: evidence from systematic reviews. Part II. Recommendations for prevention and treatment, and research agenda. Acta Anaesthesiologica Scandinavica 45: 14–19.

Waxler B. (2005) Primer of postoperative pruritus for anesthesiologists. Anesthesiology 103: 168–78.

White P. (2005) Effect of low-dose droperidol on the QT interval during and after general anesthesia. Anesthesiology 102: 1101–5.

Woodhouse A, Ward ME, Mather LE. (1999) Intrasubject variability in postoperative patient-controlled analgesia (PCA): is the patient equally satisfied with morphine, pethidine and fentanyl? Pain 80: 545–53.

Pharmacology of local anesthetic drugs

Chapter contents

Cocaine was first introduced into medical practice in 1884 by Koller, who described its use for topical anesthesia of the cornea. This was followed by its use in nerve conduction blockade and local infiltration anesthesia. In 1899 Bier reported on the application of cocaine in spinal anesthesia.

The toxicity of cocaine and its brief duration of action limited its usefulness in surgical practice and led to a search for less toxic and longer-acting substances. The synthesis of procaine by Einhorn in 1905 and of lidocaine (lignocaine) by Löfgren and Lundqvist in 1943 heralded the development of local anesthetic drugs in common use today.

Mechanism of action

Local anesthetic drugs block the generation and conduction of nerve impulses within the peripheral and central nervous systems. This requires the initiation and subsequent propagation of an action potential, a process that involves the opening of sodium channels in the nerve cell membrane. This leads to a massive flow of sodium ions from the outside to the inside of the cell membrane, which depolarizes the membrane. Immediately after depolarization the membrane is actively repolarized by ion pumps, back to its resting membrane potential. It is then available for another depolarization.

Local anesthetic drugs block sodium channels in the cell membrane, thereby preventing the influx of sodium ions, the generation of action potentials and the conduction of nerve impulses (see Figure 5.1). The blockade of sodium channels explains not only the effects, but also the adverse effects of local anesthetics; these adverse effects occur primarily as a result of interference with the generation of action potentials and conduction in the heart and central nervous system (CNS).

Local anesthetics do not have a specific analgesic effect, but can block all nerve conduction in all sensory and motor fibers. The degree of blockade is dependent on a number of factors. It is therefore useful to look briefly at the different types of nerve fiber and their size and function (Box 5.1).

It is commonly believed that smaller-diameter nerve fibers are more easily blocked than those with a larger diameter, but diameter alone is not important. The ease with which a nerve fiber is blocked by a local anesthetic drug depends also on its *critical blocking length* (the length of nerve fiber that must be exposed to the drug in order block conduction); this is

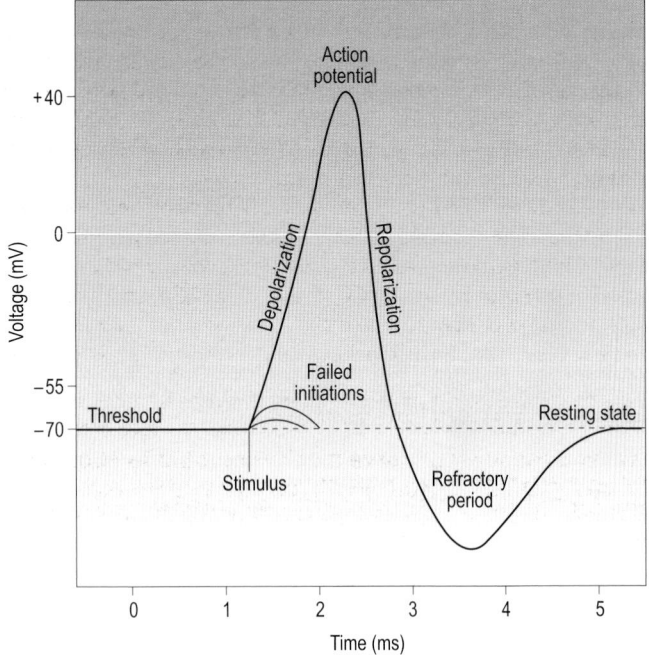

Figure 5.1 The changes in membrane potential during an action potential and during failed initiations due to local anesthetic effects.

Box 5.1

Nerve fiber class, size and function

Class	Size	Function
Myelinated fibers		
A-alpha (Aα)	Largest	Motor, proprioception (position sense)
A-beta (Aβ)		Touch, pressure
A-gamma (Aγ)		Muscle spindle tone
A-delta (Aδ)		Pain, temperature, touch
B		Preganglionic autonomic (sympathetic)
Unmyelinated fibers		
C	Smallest	Pain/temperature
		Postganglionic autonomic (sympathetic)

shorter for unmyelinated than for myelinated fibers. Another factor is the *accessibility* of nerve membrane-binding sites to the blocking agent.

However, smaller-diameter fibers have the smallest critical blocking lengths and are more easily accessed and blocked by local anesthetic solutions. Nerve blockade is also *frequency dependent*, i.e. active nerve fibers are more easily blocked than inactive ones.

The onset and regression of a nerve block usually progresses according to the order shown in Box 5.2, but this may vary a little between patients and different drugs. Note that B fibers tend to be blocked before C fibers. This is probably because C fibers are usually arranged in Remak bundles, which may hamper the diffusion of local anesthetic solutions, and/or because the critical blocking length of B fibers is quite short.

Box 5.2

Onset and recovery of nerve block according to fiber size

	Order of onset	Order of recovery
First	B	Aα
	C, Aδ	Aβ
	Aγ	Aγ
	Aβ	C, Aδ
Last	Aα	B

Overall, sympathetic blockade, with a feeling of warmth reported by the patient and vasodilation observed by the operator, usually occurs first, followed by block of nociception and temperature sensation. Motor block is commonly the last to be complete.

As the effect of a nerve block is wearing off, recovery of movement (larger fibers) may precede recovery of sensory function and pain perception or sympathetic nerve function (smaller fibers). This is of particular importance following epidural or spinal anesthesia, when a patient may have normal motor function yet may have incomplete return of sensation, and a residual sympathetic block that could lead to postural (orthostatic) hypotension.

The higher the concentration of local anesthetic solution used, the more likely nerves of all sizes are to be blocked. Low concentrations can therefore be used in an attempt to block the smaller sensory fibers only (*differential nerve block*). This approach is commonly utilized with local anesthetic infusions given via epidural and peripheral nerve catheters, and is aimed to enable the patient to move the affected limb and walk normally while still receiving good pain relief. However, there may be differences in response due to interindividual variability and catheter position, and some patients may still have some degree of motor block even with the lower concentrations. Therefore, every patient with an epidural infusion should be assessed before walking is allowed.

Blockade of sympathetic nerve fibers may also be present, which may be beneficial after peripheral vascular or plastic surgery as it leads to increased blood flow. However, with epidural analgesia, postural hypotension remains a potential risk.

Efficacy of local anesthetic drugs

The potency and hence the efficacy of a local anesthetic is related primarily to its lipid solubility, whereas the duration of action is dependent to some extent on the degree of protein binding at the site of action, as well as factors that affect the removal of the drug from the site, such as the blood supply and the addition of vasoconstrictors.

The speed of onset of a nerve block depends on the physicochemical properties of the specific anesthetic drug used. The most important determinant is the pKa value, which in relation to the physiological pH determines the local availability of un-ionized free drug. A higher pKa is associated with a slower onset of action under physiological pH conditions; this can be improved by increasing the concentration of local anesthetic, or by increasing the pH of the solution or nearby tissues.

Just as opioids have equianalgesic doses, local anesthetic drugs given in equal volumes have equieffective anesthetic concentrations (Box 5.3).

Box 5.3

Equieffective anesthetic concentrations

Local anesthetic drug	Concentration (%)
Lidocaine (lignocaine)	1
Bupivacaine	0.25
Ropivacaine	0.25–0.35*
Levobupivacaine	0.25
Prilocaine	1
Chloroprocaine	2
Procaine	2
Mepivacaine	1
Etidocaine	0.5

*Results vary according to different studies.

However, the situation here is more complicated, as the total dose administered is also an important determinant of effect. The issue of relative potency becomes even more complex when lower doses and concentrations are used to provide analgesic rather than anesthetic effects for patients in labor or during the postoperative period.

Titration studies carried out to determine a minimum local anesthetic concentration (MLAC) – an analogy to an effective dose in 50% of patients (ED_{50}) for other drugs – found potency differences between bupivacaine and ropivacaine, for example. The clinical relevance of such findings is under discussion, as in clinical practice an effect in more than 50% of patients is mandatory.

Adverse effects of local anesthetic drugs

The adverse effects that may follow the administration of a local anesthetic agent can be a result of the physiological consequences of blocking the function of certain nerves, local tissue toxicity or systemic toxicity.

Physiological effects

Physiological effects are most commonly due to blockade of the sympathetic nervous system and are most relevant after epidural and spinal anesthesia or analgesia (see Chapter 9).

Local tissue toxicity

All local anesthetics are neurotoxic in high concentrations. In vitro, lidocaine (lignocaine) and tetracaine have been shown to be neurotoxic even in concentrations used clinically. However, in clinical practice, local anesthetic agents have an enviable safety record with regard to neurotoxicity and rarely, if ever, cause localized nerve damage. An exception has been a series of reports of cauda equina syndrome following intrathecal administration of local anesthetics, in particular hyperbaric lidocaine administered via spinal microcatheters. These cases reflect the effects of high concentrations of local anesthetic accumulating near lumbosacral nerve roots due to insufficient mixing with cerebrospinal fluid when given by these very thin catheters. These catheters are no longer used, or are used only with restricted doses.

Over the last 15 years another phenomenon has been described which was initially thought to be a result of neurotoxicity. This was originally named 'transient radicular irritation', but more recently the terms 'transient neurologic symptoms' (TNS) and 'transient lumbar pain' have been coined. It presents as a temporary pain syndrome affecting the gluteal region and the lower extremities following spinal anesthesia, in particular when lidocaine has been used. However, patients describe pain only and have no neurological symptoms or abnormalities on testing. Although this has also been attributed to other local anesthetics, lidocaine has the highest propensity to cause TNS, and the continued use of lidocaine for spinal anesthesia has therefore been questioned.

The cause of TNS remains unclear; the addition of glucose, the hyperosmolarity and the hyperbaricity of the solution do not contribute to the incidence. It is of interest that surgical position is a contributing factor to the risk of TNS: potential causes under discussion are musculoskeletal strain and stretching of the sciatic nerve.

Other reports of neurotoxicity relate to the adverse effects of antioxidants, preservatives and excipients that may be added to local anesthetic solutions. For example, motor and sensory nerve deficits following subarachnoid administration of chloroprocaine were reported and thought to be due to the presence of the antioxidant sodium bisulfite in the solution. The sodium bisulfite was replaced with ethylenediaminetetra-acetic acid (EDTA) in later formulations, but since then reports of back pain have occurred.

Local anesthetics can also cause skeletal muscle toxicity. In vitro, intramuscular injections of these drugs can result in reversible myonecrosis. In this experimental setting the extent of such damage is dose dependent and increases with repeated or continuous administration. Of all the local anesthetic agents, bupivacaine seems to be the most myotoxic. Despite these well-studied experimental myotoxic effects, cases of such complications in vivo, i.e. in patients, are exceedingly rare. The few case reports published describe myopathy and/or myonecrosis after continuous infusions into peripheral nerve sheaths, but also after infiltration of wound margins and, in particular, after eye blocks.

Systemic toxicity

High blood concentrations of local anesthetic drugs can lead to signs and symptoms of systemic toxicity. This results from the effects of local anesthetic drugs on the CNS and cardiovascular system. This can occur if an otherwise safe dose is inadvertently injected directly into a blood vessel, excessive doses of local anesthetic agents are given (by injection or long-term infusion), relatively high amounts are injected into highly vascular areas (e.g. intercostal space), or if their metabolism is reduced by severe hepatic impairment. The higher the blood concentration, the more severe the signs and symptoms (Box 5.4). Not all the signs and symptoms will necessarily occur in every patient.

A number of factors will influence the blood concentrations of local anesthetic agent reached after injection:

- *Dose of drug*: this should be appropriate for the patient and the local block procedure employed; 'recommended' or 'safe' doses may be excessive if injected directly into blood vessels or tissues with a rich vascular supply.

Box 5.4

Signs and symptoms of systemic local anesthetic toxicity

Cardiovascular depression
Respiratory arrest
Coma
Convulsions
Unconsciousness   *Increasing blood*
Drowsiness   *concentrations*
Muscular twitching
Tinnitus, visual disturbances
Circumoral numbness and numbness of tongue
Lightheadedness

- *Site of injection*: the rate of absorption of local anesthetic agents depends to a large extent on the blood supply to the area; the order, from most to least rapid, is interpleural > intercostal > caudal > epidural > brachial plexus > sciatic/femoral.
- *Vasoconstrictor*: with some local anesthetic drugs (short to medium duration, e.g. lidocaine and mepivacaine) the addition of a vasoconstrictor such as epinephrine (adrenaline) will decrease the rate of absorption of drug into the circulation, prolonging the duration of action and leading to lower blood levels for the same dose; little, if any, effect is seen if epinephrine is added to prilocaine or ropivacaine.
- *Speed of injection*: the more rapid the rate of injection the more rapid the rise in plasma concentration of the drug; in a general ward a continuous infusion of local anesthetic solution may be the safest method of administration.
- *Metabolism of the drug*: severe liver impairment can reduce the clearance of local anesthetic drugs.

These deliberations make it obvious that the current concept of a maximum recommended dose for local anesthetics has little relevance in clinical practice. New recommendations will therefore be needed that take into consideration specific sites of injection as well as patient characteristics.

Central nervous system toxicity

Signs and symptoms of CNS toxicity are generally seen at lower blood concentrations than those leading to cardiovascular toxicity. The early signs are those of CNS excitation, owing to initial blockade of inhibitory pathways. Premonitory signs of CNS toxicity are best detected by maintaining verbal contact with the patient who, as blood concentrations of the drug rise, may complain of numbness around the mouth and tongue, a feeling of lightheadedness, and ringing in the ears. Slurring of speech and muscle twitching will follow, and the patient may become drowsy. If the blood level continues to rise a generalized convulsion (usually brief) will occur, and at even higher concentrations respiratory depression and arrest will ensue.

Hypercarbia and acidosis reduce the convulsive threshold of the drug, increasing the risk of convulsions at lower blood levels. Conversely, hyperventilation will lower $Paco_2$ levels and help raise the seizure threshold, thereby shortening the duration of the seizure. Early ventilation will also help to overcome hypoxia, which enhances local anesthetic CNS toxicity.

If a patient has a generalized convulsion the main aims of treatment are to prevent cerebral and myocardial hypoxia, so oxygenation and ventilation are the first priorities. Small doses of an anticonvulsant such as midazolam, diazepam or thiopental (thiopentone) should be given intravenously by trained staff; overmedication of early signs of toxicity must be avoided. Intubation of the patient may be necessary if ventilation is difficult, the patient is apneic, or there is a need to protect the airway.

Cardiovascular toxicity

In general, higher doses are required to produce cardiovascular toxicity than CNS toxicity. However, with the more potent local anesthetic agents, bupivacaine and etidocaine, life-threatening arrhythmias (which may be resistant to treatment) have occurred without CNS signs. A CNS mechanism may contribute to this cardiotoxicity.

Local anesthetic drugs can directly affect the muscles of the heart and peripheral blood vessels, and toxicity may result in alterations to myocardial contractility, conductivity and rhythmicity. Arrhythmias caused by high systemic concentrations of local anesthetics usually involve ventricular ectopy, which may progress to more malignant arrhythmias such as ventricular tachycardia, *torsades de pointes* and ventricular fibrillation, but can also present as conduction delay, complete heart block, sinus arrest or asystole.

Acidosis, hypercapnia and hypoxia markedly enhance the cardiotoxicity of local anesthetic agents. It is therefore vital to treat any convulsion promptly and effectively.

Treatment of malignant arrhythmias caused by local anesthetic overdose should follow established guidelines for advanced cardiac life support, including early defibrillation and the use of the antiarrhythmic amiodarone. Vasopressin might be a more appropriate vasoconstrictor than epinephrine, which can exacerbate arrhythmias induced by local anesthetics. Novel, more mechanistically based approaches that show promise include the use of lipid or insulin/glucose/potassium infusions.

Bupivacaine in particular can lead to severe cardiotoxicity at an early stage, and this is often refractory to aggressive and appropriate resuscitation, including defibrillation. Such cases require prolonged maintenance of resuscitation efforts (sometimes necessitating temporary extracorporeal circulation) to avoid fatalities. As outlined below, the enantiomer-specific long-lasting local anesthetics ropivacaine and levobupivacaine offer safety advantages. The cardiotoxicity of these agents is usually preceded by premonitory CNS symptoms and is less severe and easier to treat than that caused by bupivacaine.

Commonly used local anesthetic drugs

Local anesthetic agents are classified according to the nature of the linkage between the lipid-soluble and water-soluble parts of the molecule; the two types of linkage are *amides* and *esters* (see Figure 5.2). The clinical differences between the two involve the mechanisms by which they are metabolized and their potential for producing allergic reactions. Representatives of the two classes are discussed below and listed in Box 5.5.

Esters

Ester local anesthetic drugs are metabolized in plasma (and to a lesser extent the liver) by pseudocholinesterases, hence their half-lives in the circulation are shorter than those of the amide local anesthetics. These drugs have a greater potential to cause allergic reactions, as they are metabolized to para-amino benzoic acid (PABA), which acts as a hapten. They are also less stable in solution than amide local anesthetics. For these reasons they are not widely used, are no longer registered in many countries, and are now more of historical interest. In particular, they play no role in the treatment of acute pain.

Cocaine

Cocaine has a number of actions in addition to its ability to block conduction of nerve impulses. It causes general stimulation of the CNS and blocks reuptake of catecholamines at adrenergic nerve endings, thus

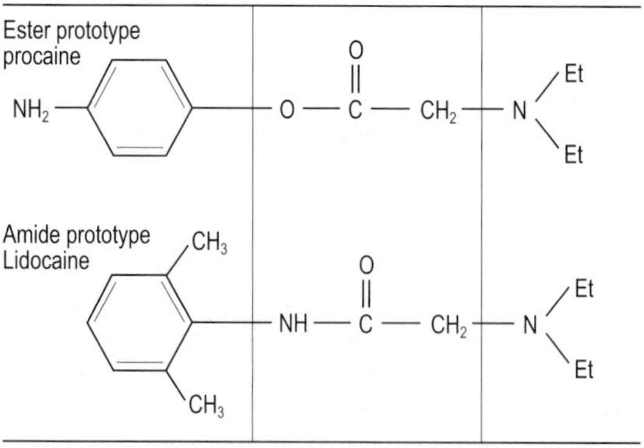

Figure 5.2 Prototype structures of ester and amide local anesthetics.

Box 5.5

Classes of local anesthetic drug

Amides	Esters
Lidocaine (lignocaine)	Procaine
Bupivacaine	Chloroprocaine
Ropivacaine	Cocaine
Levobupivacaine	Tetracaine (amethocaine)
Mepivacaine	Benzocaine
Etidocaine	
Prilocaine	
Dibucaine (cinchocaine)	

potentiating the effects of sympathetic nervous system stimulation. These changes can lead to euphoria and a feeling of wellbeing, restlessness, excitement, tachycardia, peripheral vasoconstriction, hypertension, arrhythmias, myocardial ischemia and convulsions. Because of its potential for toxicity, cocaine is now restricted to use as a topical anesthetic agent, usually in surgery involving the nose or preceding nasal endotracheal intubation, where its local vasoconstrictor effect helps to shrink the nasal mucosa and reduce bleeding. Doses should be kept within recommended limits to avoid the risk of side effects.

Tetracaine (amethocaine)

Tetracaine is used primarily for spinal anesthesia.

Procaine

Procaine was the first synthetic local anesthetic agent introduced into clinical practice. Its use is now confined mainly to local infiltration.

Chloroprocaine

Because of its rapid onset, rapid metabolism and short duration of action, chloroprocaine has been used primarily in obstetric epidural analgesia or regional anesthetic techniques for day surgery. Neurotoxicity, with motor and sensory deficits, has followed accidental subarachnoid injection; the sodium bisulfite antioxidant in the anesthetic solution was implicated. The bisulfite was replaced by EDTA in later formulations, but this has been followed by reports of muscle spasm and backache.

Amides

Amide local anesthetic drugs are metabolized in the liver and the elimination half-lives vary from about 1.5 hours to 3.5 hours. These drugs rarely, if ever, cause true allergic reactions, although patients may be allergic to the antioxidants and preservatives contained in some local anesthetic solutions. These were a particular problem with multidose vials, which have been discontinued in most countries. Some patients reporting an 'allergy' to these drugs may have experienced effects due to the systemic absorption of epinephrine, or an allergic reaction to an ester local anesthetic, or had a vasovagal response to the injection.

A differentiation between the short-acting amides (e.g. lidocaine) and the long-acting amide agents (bupivacaine, levobupivacaine and ropivacaine), which are most often used for continuous maintenance of regional analgesia, is clinically useful.

Lidocaine (lignocaine)

Lidocaine is the most widely used short-acting local anesthetic worldwide. Absorption can be reduced (and hence duration of action increased and the risk of toxicity decreased) by the addition of epinephrine to the solution. Although often used to establish regional and local anesthetic blocks for operative procedures, it is not commonly used in the ongoing management of acute pain. Reasons for this include the development of acute tolerance and tachyphylaxis, as well as the propensity to cause a greater degree of motor block than the long-acting local anesthetics.

Lidocaine is available in a number of preparations: ointments, jelly, topical solutions including a spray, and formulations for injection. It has also been administered by nebulizer to obtain topical anesthesia of the upper airway, and intravenously for the treatment of cardiac arrhythmias and neuropathic pain (see Chapter 12).

A mixture of lidocaine and prilocaine (2.5% of each), called EMLA cream (eutectic mixture of local anesthetics), can be used as a topical local anesthetic agent for skin. Applied under an occlusive dressing or as a patch, it takes 30–60 minutes to have its full effect. It has been used prior to the insertion of intravenous cannulae or other needles (especially in children), and for local procedures such as superficial skin surgery and skin grafting.

A topical lidocaine patch is also available in some countries and has been used in the management of pain due to acute herpes zoster and postherpetic neuralgia.

Bupivacaine

Bupivacaine (a long-acting drug) is commonly used for the management of acute pain outside the operating room. In the ward setting, low doses and administration by infusion minimize the risk of toxicity; infusion solutions of 0.125% bupivacaine for the provision of continuous epidural and of 0.25% for continuous regional analgesia are commercially available in a number of countries.

As outlined above, bupivacaine is more cardiotoxic than other local anesthetic drugs, and any cardiovascular collapse that does occur may be more difficult to treat. The addition of epinephrine has little effect on the duration of action of the drug, including when used epidurally.

Bupivacaine has one asymmetric C atom and therefore shows stereoisomerism. It is a racemic mixture of two enantiomers, $S-(-)$ and $R-(+)$, which have the same structural formula but a different three-dimensional configuration of atoms; the two molecules are therefore not superimposable – similar to mirror images or our two hands. This leads to different biological activities of the two enantiomers, with $R-(+)$ being more toxic to the heart and CNS.

In response to these findings, the enantiomer-specific local anesthetics ropivacaine, and more recently levobupivacaine, have been released. They have a lower potential for CNS and cardiotoxicity, which has been confirmed in animal studies and for surrogate outcomes of toxicity in healthy volunteers. Furthermore, resuscitation of dogs showing toxicity was significantly more successful when the enantiomer-specific agents were given. These results are confirmed by the currently published case reports of accidental toxic overdoses, which suggest better outcomes and response to resuscitation after ropivacaine and levobupivacaine than after bupivacaine.

Ropivacaine

Ropivacaine is the $S-(-)$ enantiomer of the propyl analog of bupivacaine. It is said to have a potency comparable to that of bupivacaine, with a similar onset, duration and degree of sensory block when given in equivalent doses, although in some studies it appears to be less potent. Another advantage over bupivacaine is said to be a greater differential block (less motor block for the same degree of sensory block); however, in acute pain management, when low concentrations of bupivacaine are commonly given by infusion, the difference in degree of motor blockade between the two drugs is not always apparent. A 0.2% solution for infusion is commercially available in a number of countries.

Levobupivacaine

Levobupivacaine is the S−(−) enantiomer of bupivacaine. Compared with racemic bupivacaine, levobupivacaine has similar anesthetic properties but, like ropivacaine, a lower potential for cardiotoxicity, and therefore offers similar advantages.

Mepivacaine

Mepivacaine has a similar anesthetic profile to lidocaine, with a relatively rapid onset and a moderate duration of action. Unlike lidocaine, mepivacaine is effective as a topical agent only in large doses, and should not be used for this indication.

Prilocaine

Prilocaine has a similar clinical profile to lidocaine, but is the least toxic of the amide local anesthetic drugs. This makes it a suitable choice for intravenous regional anesthesia (Bier's block).

The initial step in the metabolism of prilocaine forms orthotoluidine. The administration of large doses may lead to the accumulation of this metabolite, which in turn leads to an increase in the oxidation of hemoglobin to methemoglobin. If the level of methemoglobin becomes excessive, the patient may appear cyanotic. This metabolic toxicity limits the use of prilocaine in anemic patients and leads to the recommendation to avoid repeat injections or infusions, thereby limiting its use in acute pain therapy.

Dibucaine (cinchocaine)

Dibucaine is widely used to provide topical analgesia, e.g. in creams and ointments. The injectable preparation is used primarily for spinal analgesia.

Etidocaine

Etidocaine is as long-acting as bupivacaine and has been associated with similar problems with respect to cardiotoxicity. It is noted for its profound motor blockade and is therefore not used to provide analgesia.

Key points

Evidence level

I Continuous perineural infusions of lidocaine (lignocaine) result in less effective analgesia and more motor block than long-acting local anesthetic agents

II There are no consistent differences between ropivacaine, levobupivacaine and bupivacaine in terms of quality of analgesia or motor blockade when given in low doses for regional analgesia

II Cardiovascular and central nervous system effects of the stereospecific isomers ropivacaine and levobupivacaine are less severe than those resulting from racemic bupivacaine

---

Clinical practice points

Case reports following accidental overdose with ropivacaine and bupivacaine suggest that resuscitation is likely to be more successful with ropivacaine

Reproduced with permission from Acute Pain Management: Scientific Evidence ANZCA and FPM (2005)

References and further reading

Australian and New Zealand College of Anaesthetists, Faculty of Pain Medicine. Acute Pain Management: Scientific Evidence, 2nd edn. Melbourne: Australian and New Zealand College of Anaesthetists (2005). Also available online at: *http://www.anzca.edu. au/publications/acutepain.htm* and *http://www7.health.gov.au/nhmrc / publications/synopses/cp104syn.htm*

Casati A, Putzu M. (2005) Bupivacaine, levobupivacaine and ropivacaine: are they clinically different? Best Practice in Research and Clinical Anaesthesiology 19: 247–68.

Cox B, Durieux ME, Marcus MA. (2003) Toxicity of local anaesthetics. Best Practice and Research in Clinical Anaesthesiology 17: 111–36.

De Jong RH. (1994) Local anesthetics. St Louis: Mosby.

Mather LE, Copeland SE, Ladd LA. (2005) Acute toxicity of local anesthetics: underlying pharmacokinetic and pharmacodynamic concepts. Regional Anesthesia Pain Medicine 30: 553–66.

McClure JH. (1996) Ropivacaine. British Journal of Anaesthesia 76: 300–7.

McLeod GA, Burke D. (2001) Levobupivacaine. Anaesthesia 56: 331–41.

Mulroy MF. (2002) Systemic toxicity and cardiotoxicity from local anesthetics: incidence and preventive measures. Regional Anesthesia Pain Medicine 27: 556–61.

Pollock JE. (2003) Neurotoxicity of intrathecal local anaesthetics and transient neurological symptoms. Best Practice in Research and Clinical Anaesthesiology 17: 471–84.

Serpell M. (2003) Clinical pharmacology – local anesthetics. In: Rowbotham D, Macintyre P, eds. Clinical pain management: acute volume. London: Arnold.

Sidebotham DA, Schug SA. (1997) Stereochemistry in anaesthesia. Clinical and Experimental Pharmacology and Physiology 24: 126–30.

Thomas JM, Schug SA. (1999) Recent advances in the pharmacokinetics of local anaesthetics. Long-acting amide enantiomers and continuous infusions. Clinical Pharmacokinetics 36: 67–83.

Weinberg GL. (2002) Current concepts in resuscitation of patients with local anesthetic cardiac toxicity. Regional Anesthesia Pain Medicine 27: 568–75.

Zaric D, Chistiansen C, Pace NL et al. (2005) Transient neurological symptoms after spinal anesthesia with lidocaine versus other local anesthetics: a systematic review of randomized controlled trials. Anesthesia and Analgesia 100: 1811–16.

Zink, W, Graf BM. (2004) Local anesthetic myotoxicity. Regional Anesthesia Pain Medicine 29: 333–40.

Non-opioid and adjuvant analgesic agents

CHAPTER

6

Chapter contents

Drugs other than opioids and local anesthetic agents may be used in the treatment of acute pain, either as the sole agent or as adjuvant medication. Such drugs include the non-opioid analgesics, i.e. simple paracetamol (acetaminophen) and the non-steroidal anti-inflammatory drugs (including the subgroup of selective COX-2 inhibitors – coxibs), the inhalational agent nitrous oxide, and a large group of drugs that are commonly called adjuvant analgesic agents or co-analgesics. A number of these (e.g. antidepressants, anticonvulsants) are used primarily in the management of neuropathic pain (see Chapter 12).

Paracetamol (acetaminophen)

Although paracetamol is often classified as an NSAID, this is incorrect, as it is devoid of anti-inflammatory activity. Paracetamol is exclusively an analgesic and antipyretic agent, and as such does not cause gastrointestinal ulceration or bleeding.

The development of paracetamol began with the discovery of the fever-lowering effect of acetanilide, a finding that resulted in the development of phenacetin by Bayer. Its active metabolite, paracetamol, was first used clinically by von Mehring in 1893. Paracetamol is one of the most widely used drugs worldwide.

Mechanism of action

Despite its common use and long history, uncertainty about the mechanism of action of paracetamol continues. It has no known endogenous binding sites and, unlike NSAIDs, does not inhibit peripheral cyclo-oxygenase activity. Current hypotheses suggest a central effect leading to its antipyretic and antinociceptive properties. Antipyresis may result from inhibition of prostaglandin synthesis in the hypothalamus; the antinociceptive mechanism of action is even less well understood.

It has been suggested that paracetamol inhibits central COX-2 activity (COX-2 is an isoform of cyclo-oxygenase – see next section). However, there is ongoing discussion about its inhibitory effect on another isoenzyme, COX-3, which is a variant of COX-2 and highly sensitive to inhibition by paracetamol. Other hypotheses propose that paracetamol modulates the serotonergic (5-HT) anti-nociceptive system, has an antagonistic effect on the NMDA receptor, or has a mechanism of action related to nitric oxide. None of these hypotheses has been confirmed, and the definitive mechanism of action underlying the analgesic effect of paracetamol remains unknown.

Clinical efficacy and use

Clinically, paracetamol is a very useful analgesic. Worldwide it has become the first choice for pain relief across a wide range of indications and a wide range of patient ages. Reasons for this include its relative effectiveness in many pain conditions, its high tolerability, even for patients in whom other non-opioid drugs are contraindicated, and the minimal risk of serious adverse effects.

Paracetamol is usually given orally or rectally. After oral administration and absorption from the small bowel, peak plasma concentrations are reached within about an hour. Time to peak plasma concentration and bioavailability are much less reliable when the rectal route is used.

The use of paracetamol has been facilitated by the introduction of an intravenous preparation, now available in many countries as 1000 mg paracetamol in a 100 mL infusion bottle. This is replacing *propacetamol*, a 'prodrug' which is rapidly hydrolyzed by plasma esterases to paracetamol but which causes significant irritation and thrombophlebitis at the site of injection. Intravenous administration results in higher CNS concentrations of paracetamol and better analgesia than the oral and rectal routes.

Co-administration of an NSAID with paracetamol may significantly improve its pain-relieving effects, as will combination with various opioids, including codeine, tramadol and oxycodone. The addition of paracetamol to opioid treatment regimens results in 'opioid sparing'.

The discussion about a reasonable therapeutic dose continues. Although a dose limit of 4 g/day for adults is often suggested, higher doses may be appropriate in some settings. For limited periods at least, most adults with normal body weight and in whom there is no contraindication may be best treated with 1 g 4-hourly up to a maximum dose of 6 g/day. Chronic medication should continue with 1 g 6-hourly, i.e. 4 g/day.

Paracetamol should be regarded as the first-line analgesic for mild to moderate pain and as an important component of multimodal analgesia in the treatment of moderate and severe pain.

Adverse effects

Many misconceptions about the risks of taking paracetamol have resulted from the well-known fact that a major overdose can lead to severe and sometimes fatal liver damage. However, taken in suggested therapeutic doses, paracetamol is well tolerated by most patients and has minimal adverse effects.

Most of the drug is excreted by the kidney after glucuronide and sulfate conjugation in the liver. Hepatotoxicity following overdose is caused by *N*-acetyl-*p*-benzoquinone imine (NAPQI), a metabolite of paracetamol which is highly reactive and can lead to hepatic necrosis. However, NAPQI is normally inactivated by combination with glutathione and then metabolized to harmless compounds that undergo renal excretion. Excessive doses of paracetamol may exhaust the liver's glutathione stores; NAPQI can then cause dose-related liver damage. It has been suggested that patients who have low levels of glutathione (e.g. associated with starvation, malnutrition, HIV, chronic liver disease and regular high alcohol intake) may be more susceptible to paracetamol-associated hepatotoxicty. However, it may be that neither alcohol consumption nor nutrition places patients at increased risk, as long as recommended doses of paracetamol are used. Overdoses in such patients may result in a more severe hepatotoxicity.

Renal toxicity, historically linked to a prodrug, phenacetin, rarely occurs with paracetamol and it is recommended for use in patients with renal impairment.

Paracetamol hypersensitivity and allergies are unlikely. In patients with the rare glucose-6-phosphate dehydrogenase (G6PD) deficiency it can lead to hemolysis.

Non-selective non-steroidal anti-inflammatory drugs

The analgesic and anti-inflammatory properties of the bark of the willow and other plants have been known for centuries. The active ingredient in willow bark is *salicin* and was described in the 19th century. Subsequently, the chemist Hoffmann, trying to improve the gastric tolerability of salicylic acid for his father, synthesized acetylic–salicylic acid, the well-known aspirin. Aspirin became the prototype of non-steroidal anti-inflammatory drugs (NSAIDs). Attempts to improve this compound led to the many NSAIDs now available worldwide and the subsequent development of the COX-2 inhibitors (coxibs). From a practical point of view it is useful to look at NSAIDs and coxibs separately.

Mechanism of action

NSAIDs exhibit a spectrum of analgesic, anti-inflammatory, antiplatelet and antipyretic actions, although the degree to which these are seen may vary between drugs. In 1971 Vane, who won a Nobel Prize for his discovery, identified the mechanism of action as the inhibition of the enzyme cyclo-oxygenase. This enzyme metabolizes arachidonic acid to a large number of eicosanoids, including prostaglandins, prostacyclins and thromboxane A_2. This mechanism of action also explains the wide range of adverse effects of NSAIDs, as the eicosanoids have protective homeostatic functions in the intestinal mucosa and the kidney, and are linked to platelet function.

The anti-inflammatory effect is related to the reduction of prostaglandins such as PGE_2 and prostacyclin, which act as mediators of inflammation. The analgesic effect is the result of decreased prostaglandin synthesis in the periphery, leading to decreased sensitization of nociceptors. In addition, the inhibition of cyclo-oxygenase in the CNS reduces the formation of prostaglandins in the spinal cord and the brain, and thereby central sensitization. The antipyretic effect is the result of a decrease in prostaglandin concentrations in the hypothalamus, which increase in response to the inflammatory pyrogen interleukin-1 (IL-1).

The discovery of two isoforms of cyclo-oxygenase, COX-1 and COX-2, led to the rapid development of a series of COX-2 selective inhibitors which were marketed with great success, as they were initially thought to be devoid of many of the common adverse effects associated with the classic NSAIDs (see below).

Clinical efficacy and use

Non-steroidal anti-inflammatory drugs may be used as the sole method of treatment for mild to moderate pain, but in most patients are not sufficiently effective as the sole agent after major surgery or injury, when they are best used in combination with other analgesics such as opioids. They can, however, lead to better analgesia than lower-potency opioids such as codeine and propoxyphene.

When combined with opioids, NSAIDs may enhance the quality of analgesia. They may also lead to a 20–40% reduction in opioid requirements (i.e. they are 'opioid sparing') and a reduction in the incidence or severity of opioid-related adverse effects. Similarly, when NSAIDs are used *instead* of opioids, a significant reduction in side effects is seen.

There is a 'ceiling effect' to the analgesia produced by NSAIDs, when further increases in dose do not result in additional pain relief but may instead result in an increase in adverse effects. There appears to be little if any difference in analgesic efficacy between the different NSAIDs, although differences may exist in their anti-inflammatory activity and in the incidence of side effects. Although concurrent use of two NSAIDs is not usually recommended, pain relief is improved by the combination of paracetamol with an NSAID.

Most NSAIDs are given orally or rectally. After oral administration they are rapidly absorbed from the upper gastrointestinal tract, primarily from the stomach; peak plasma concentrations are usually reached in about 2 hours. Some (e.g. ketorolac, tenoxicam and diclofenac) can be given by injection. Oral administration is very effective and there is little evidence that other routes offer significant advantages in terms of analgesic efficacy or side effects; however, parenteral administration permits their use in patients unable to take oral medications.

Most NSAIDs are metabolized in the liver and their metabolites excreted by the kidney. Clearance is reduced in elderly patients and in those with renal disease. Most NSAIDs have half-lives of 2–3 hours, although some, such as piroxicam and tenoxicam, are much longer (50–60 hours), enabling these drugs to be given just once a day. The NSAIDs with longer half-lives may be associated with a higher incidence of adverse effects.

Precautions and contraindications

Before NSAIDs are prescribed, reference should be made to the appropriate product information sheet for each drug. Precautions, contraindications, suggested doses and duration of therapy, potential drug interactions and permitted routes of administration may vary between different drugs and different countries.

An evidence-based report by the Royal College of Anaesthetists considered the use of NSAIDs in the postoperative period and suggested certain precautions and contraindications. These are summarized in Box 6.1.

Box 6.1

Possible precautions and contraindications to the use of NSAIDs for acute pain management

NSAIDs should be avoided in the following clinical situations:

- Pre-existing renal impairment (elevated plasma creatinine levels)
- Hyperkalemia
- Dehydration, hypovolemia or hypotension from any cause
- Cardiac failure
- Severe liver dysfunction
- Uncontrolled hypertension
- Aspirin-induced asthma
- History of gastrointestinal bleeding or ulceration
- Known hypersensitivity to aspirin or other NSAIDs

NSAIDs should be used with caution in the following clinical situations:

- Impaired hepatic function, diabetes, bleeding or coagulation disorders, vascular disease
- Operations where there is a high risk of intraoperative hemorrhage (e.g. cardiac, major vascular and hepatobiliary surgery)
- Operations where an absence of bleeding is important (e.g. eye surgery, neurosurgery and cosmetic surgery)
- Other forms of asthma
- Concurrent use of other NSAIDs (except paracetamol), ACE inhibitors, potassium-sparing diuretics, anticoagulants, methotrexate, ciclosporin (cyclosporine) and antibiotics such as gentamicin
- Children less than 16 years old
- Pregnant and lactating women
- Advanced age (renal impairment is likely in patients older than 65 years, even if creatinine levels are normal)

Many perioperative factors may adversely affect renal blood flow and it may be wise to delay the administration of NSAIDs until the postoperative period and until the patient is normovolemic and normotensive. If a patient is already receiving an NSAID it should be discontinued if there is any increase in plasma urea or creatinine levels, or if urine output is low.

Data from the guidelines of the Royal College of Anaesthetists, 1998.

Adverse effects

The NSAIDs can produce a variety of undesirable adverse effects, so the potential risk of using these drugs should always be weighed against the possible benefits. The comments below refer to the commonly used NSAIDs that show both COX-1 and COX-2 inhibition, although the degree of inhibition of each isoenzyme may vary between drugs.

Gastrointestinal

Reductions in prostaglandin levels by inhibition of COX-1 may lead to erosions of the gastrointestinal mucosa, especially in the stomach. This is due to a reduction in the prostaglandin-mediated protective functions of mucus production, maintenance of mucosal blood flow, and inhibition of gastric acid secretion. Thus, the problem will not be avoided if the drugs are given parenterally or by the rectal route. The benefit of prophylaxis against gastric effects is unclear. Prostaglandin analogs (e.g. misoprostol) and proton pump inhibitors (e.g. omeprazole) are more effective than H_2 antagonists (e.g. cimetidine, ranitidine) at reducing the incidence of these side effects.

Gastric irritation, dyspepsia and ulceration (which may be silent in approximately 50% of patients until a bleed or perforation occurs) may develop at any time, even with short-term treatment. The risk of gastrointestinal side effects increases with long-term treatment, increasing age, alcohol, history of peptic ulcer disease and/or gastric bleeding, high doses, and concurrent use of anticoagulants (including heparin used for thromboprophylaxis) or steroids. Ibuprofen and diclofenac appear to have one of the lowest incidences of gastrointestinal side effects; piroxicam and ketorolac are associated with the highest.

Other gastrointestinal complications include the development of esophagitis (in particular after intake of aspirin), a diffuse intestinal inflammation known as NSAID enteropathy, and colitis.

Renal

In patients in whom the effective circulating blood volume is reduced (e.g. as a result of hypovolemia, dehydration, hypotension, sepsis or excessive use of diuretics) or in those with congestive cardiac failure or hepatic cirrhosis, vasodilatory renal prostaglandins are released in order to maintain renal perfusion. Renal toxicity of NSAIDs is the result of COX-1 and COX-2 inhibition, as both isoenzymes produce vasodilatory prostaglandins that help to maintain renal blood flow and glomerular filtration rate. Pre-existing renal impairment will increase the risk of renal complications. It should be noted that elderly patients often have reduced renal function even though serum creatinine levels appear normal. Concurrent administration of some other drugs may also increase the risk of renal problems with NSAIDs. These include angiotensin-converting enzyme (ACE) inhibitors, potassium-sparinge diuretics, aminoglycoside antibiotics, methotrexate and ciclosporin (cyclosporine).

Acute postoperative renal failure due to NSAIDs has been reported even in healthy young patients. Many perioperative factors may adversely affect renal blood flow, and in some cases it may be wise to delay the administration of NSAIDs until the postoperative period and until the patients is normovolemic and normotensive. However, this does not mean that NSAIDs should not be given to adults with normal preoperative renal function, as supported by a recent meta-analysis. If a patient is already receiving an NSAID, it should be discontinued if there is any increase in plasma urea or creatinine, or if urine output is low.

Non-steroidal anti-inflammatory drugs can cause sodium, potassium and water retention, which may lead to edema in some patients and may reduce the effectiveness of antihypertensive therapy. Interstitial nephritis and nephrotic syndrome have also been reported in association with NSAID use.

Platelet function and bleeding times

Aggregation of platelets depends on thromboxane A_2. As the formation of thromboxane A_2 is reduced by NSAID-induced inhibition of COX-1, bleeding times may be prolonged. This may increase the risk of perioperative blood loss in some situations and leads to a higher reoperation rate for bleeding after tonsillectomy.

Aspirin is particularly effective in inhibiting platelet function as it inhibits COX *irreversibly* and effectively prolongs bleeding time for the life of the platelet (4–8 days). Recovery depends on the production of new platelets. Other NSAIDs *reversibly* inhibit platelet COX, and the effect lasts only as long as the drug remains in the patient.

Respiratory

Aspirin-exacerbated respiratory disease (AERD) is the induction of asthma and bronchospasm that may follow NSAID administration in some patients. NSAIDs should therefore be used with caution in these patients. Up to 5–10% of adult asthmatic patients may develop AERD, and a cross-sensitivity can exist between aspirin and other NSAIDs.

Other effects

Headache, anxiety, depression, confusion, dizziness, somnolence, hypertension and cardiac failure have all been reported following the administration of NSAIDs, as have a variety of skin reactions and blood dyscrasias.

Abnormalities in liver function tests may be seen, but these are usually transient. Rarely, hepatotoxicity occurs. A specific form of hepatotoxicity is linked to Reye's syndrome. Although the cause of this remains unclear, the syndrome is associated with the intake of aspirin during a viral illness (e.g. an upper respiratory tract infection or chickenpox) in children. As well as liver failure, these children may develop cerebral inflammation and edema and the results may be fatal.

There is evidence that, by inhibiting prostaglandin synthesis, NSAIDs impair osteoblast activity. This may impair healing after spinal fusion and fractures.

NSAIDs may affect the actions of other drugs that are dependent on the kidney for excretion, such as the aminoglycoside antibiotics (e.g. gentamicin) and digoxin.

Selective COX-2 inhibitors

The discovery of two isoforms of cyclo-oxygenase, COX-1 and COX-2, rapidly resulted in the development of a new class of analgesic and anti-inflammatory drugs, the so-called selective COX-2 inhibitors or coxibs. COX-2 is found in inflammatory cells, sites of inflammation and tissue damage, the synovium of joints, endothelium and the central nervous system, and was the logical choice as the target of a new class of drug that might avoid classic NSAID-related adverse effects.

Mechanism of action

The isoenzyme COX-1 is a *constitutively* expressed cyclo-oxygenase found in the gastrointestinal tract, kidney and platelets. It maintains gastric cytoprotection, renal sodium and water balance, and normal platelet aggregation. The isoenzyme COX-2 was initially regarded only as *inducible*, by inflammatory cytokinines such as interleukins. However, it is also a constitutive enzyme in the brain, kidney, ovary, uterus and endothelium.

The discovery of a hydrophilic side pocket in the wider COX-2 isoform of the enzyme enabled the development of larger molecules with a side chain that fitted the side pocket but did not fit the COX-1 isoform.

Clinical efficacy and use

Within a very short time two initial coxibs, rofecoxib and celecoxib, were developed and marketed for use in patients with osteoarthritis and rheumatoid arthritis. Subsequently, others such as valdecoxib and its parenterally administered prodrug, parecoxib, as well as etirocoxib and lumiracoxib, became available.

Coxibs are as effective as NSAIDs for the treatment of arthritic pain and moderate to severe postoperative pain. Combined with opioids as a component of multimodal analgesia, they result in opioid sparing, improved pain relief, and a reduced incidence of adverse opioid-related effects.

Parecoxib is particularly suitable for acute pain management as it can be given as an intravenous (IV) or intramuscular (IM) injection. It provides a rapid onset of analgesia – within 10–15 minutes – which lasts 12–24 hours. Lumiracoxib is registered in a number of countries for oral use in the treatment of acute pain; celecoxib is also widely used.

Adverse effects

In the treatment of acute pain, coxibs can offer significant advantages over non-selective NSAIDs with regard to adverse effects.

Whereas even short-term use of NSAIDs (such as naproxen and ketorolac) is associated with a high incidence of gastrointestinal ulceration, the rate with parecoxib is identical to that of placebo. Coxibs do not impair platelet function and therefore do not increase the risk of postoperative bleeding, and they do not induce AERD. Animal studies and limited human studies suggest that they do not impair bone healing to the same extent as the non-selective NSAIDs. However, coxibs can have the same adverse effect on renal function and should be used with the same precautions. A comparative table of the adverse effects of NSAIDs and coxibs is provided in Box 6.2.

Box 6.2

Comparison of adverse effects with perioperative non-selective NSAID or selective coxib treatment (i.e. short-term treatment)

Adverse effect	NSAID	Coxib
Upper gastrointestinal ulcers	+	−
Bleeding	+	−
Bone healing ↓	(+)	−
Aspirin-sensitive asthma	+	−
Renal function ↓	+	+

Cardiac

The withdrawal of rofecoxib from the market in September 2004, because of an increased incidence of thrombembolic complications (i.e. myocardial infarction, stroke) associated with its long-term use, initiated debate about a potential 'class effect' of coxibs. This was based on the hypothesis that selective inhibition of the COX-2 isoform would lead to an imbalance between endothelial prostacyclin production and lack of thromboxane A_2 formation in platelets; such an imbalance could have a prothrombotic effect. However, it would appear that the increased

---

Key points

Evidence level

I Paracetamol is an effective analgesic for acute pain

I NSAIDs and COX-2 inhibitors are effective analgesics of similar efficacy for acute pain

I NSAIDs given in addition to paracetamol improve analgesia

I With careful patient selection and monitoring, the incidence of NSAID-induced perioperative renal impairment is low

I Aspirin and some NSAIDs increase the risk of perioperative bleeding after tonsillectomy

I COX-2 inhibitors and NSAIDs have similar adverse effects on renal function

I COX-2 selective inhibitors do not appear to produce bronchospasm in individuals known to have aspirin-exacerbated respiratory disease

II Paracetamol, NSAIDs and COX-2 inhibitors are valuable components of multimodal analgesia

II COX-2 inhibitors do not impair platelet function

II Short-term use of COX-2 inhibitors results in gastric ulceration rates similar to those of placebo

II Use of parecoxib followed by valdecoxib after coronary artery bypass surgery increases the incidence of cardiovascular events

---

Clinical practice points

Adverse effects of NSAIDs are significant and may limit their use

The risk of adverse renal effects of NSAIDs and COX-2 inhibitors is increased in the presence of factors such as pre-existing renal impairment, hypovolemia, hypotension, use of other nephrotoxic agents and ACE inhibitors

incidence of thrombembolic complications is a class effect of most, if not all, anti-inflammatory drugs, and not just coxibs.

The administration of parecoxib and valdecoxib after coronary bypass graft surgery has been shown to increase the incidence of cardio- and cerebrovascular events, and their use in this type of surgery is now contraindicated. This is most likely due to the unusual situation after cardiopulmonary bypass, with activation of platelets and endothelial cells combined with reperfusion injury and emboli in cardiovascular high-risk patients. Studies and meta-analyses in patients after general surgery have not identified any increased risk of such complications.

Nitrous oxide

Nitrous oxide (N_2O) is one of the oldest inhalational anesthetics available. It is not very potent, but has analgesic properties in subanesthetic concentrations.

Clinical efficacy and use

Owing to its physicochemical properties, nitrous oxide has a rapid onset and a short duration of action; some effect will be seen after four or five deep breaths. Offset of effect is also rapid, and so analgesia can only be maintained by repeated inhalations. It is therefore suitable to provide analgesia during labor and for painful procedures such as dental surgery, endoscopy, dressing changes, biopsies and venous cannulation. It will often be used in combination with opioid or other analgesic therapies. In some institutions, concerns about environmental nitrous oxide levels limit its use in general wards.

Nitrous oxide is commonly used in some countries as a combination of 50% nitrous oxide and 50% oxygen in premixed cylinders (Entonox). In other countries, the use of a mixing valve permits a variety of nitrous oxide/oxygen combinations to be given.

A one-way demand valve allows delivery of the gas when the patient inspires, providing there is an airtight fit between face and mask or mouthpiece. The technique is inherently safe, as it is self-administered: if the patient becomes too drowsy the mask will fall away from their face. As nitrous oxide causes minimal respiratory depression it can be used without the presence of medical staff, as long as unconsciousness is avoided.

Adverse effects

Air-containing spaces

Gases equilibrate across permeable membranes so that concentrations on either side become equal. Nitrous oxide equilibrates rapidly, nitrogen much more slowly. If a patient breathes a mixture containing only oxygen and nitrous oxide, the concentration of nitrous oxide in any air-containing space will rise rapidly. However, the concentration of nitrogen in that space will fall much more slowly, so that there is an overall increase in volume of the gas space. If the space cannot expand there can be a marked increase in pressure. Nitrous oxide is therefore contraindicated in patients with a pneumothorax, pneumocephalus, bowel obstruction or obstruction of the middle ear or sinus cavities, or who have had recent vitreoretinal surgery with use of gas or a recent gas embolism (e.g. divers).

Toxicity

Nitrous oxide oxidizes vitamin B_{12} and thereby inactivates the enzyme methionine synthetase, leading to depletion of vitamin B_{12}, tetrahydrofolate and methionine. Potential consequences of these effects are bone marrow and neurotoxicity.

It used to be thought that these complications might only follow prolonged or repeated administration of nitrous oxide, but the exact duration of exposure required to cause these changes is unknown. Neurotoxicity has been reported after a single, short-term exposure in susceptible patients (see below).

The clinical features resemble those of vitamin B_{12} deficiency. However, vitamin B_{12} levels may be normal, as the problem is due to a reduction in *active* vitamin B_{12} levels, not necessarily total body levels.

Bone marrow toxicity leads to megaloblastic anemia and then, in some patients, to thrombocytopenia and leukopenia. These effects are progressive, but are also reversible and preventable by the administration of folinic acid.

Neurotoxicity resulting from nitrous oxide use is rare, but it can develop rapidly and may be irreversible. The neuropathy results from decreased methionine levels and a subsequent reduction in myelin synthesis, leading to demyelination of nerves. The clinical features are similar to those seen in patients with vitamin B_{12} deficiency and subacute combined degeneration of the spinal cord, and include numbness, paresthesiae, ataxia and spasticity. The risk of this complication is significantly increased in patients with a pre-existing vitamin B_{12} deficiency (e.g. vegetarians or the elderly), when even short-term exposure to nitrous oxide can cause a severe neuropathy. The vitamin B_{12} deficiency may be subclinical, i.e. detectable only by measuring blood levels.

There is a paucity of evidence relating to the prevention or treatment of complications due to nitrous oxide-related inactivation of vitamin B_{12}. As nitrous oxide interferes with the function of vitamin B_{12}, it is possible that B_{12} supplements may not help unless given at a time remote from the administration of nitrous oxide (difficult when repeat administration is occurring). There is no clear support in the literature for the use of B_{12} supplements in this situation. Methionine supplements have been suggested for the prevention of neurological changes, but evidence for their benefit is limited. Some evidence exists for the role of folic or folinic acid (5-formyl-THF) in preventing or reversing nitrous oxide-induced bone marrow changes.

Key points

Evidence level

I Nitrous oxide is an effective analgesic during labor

II Nitrous oxide is an effective analgesic agent in a variety of other acute pain situations

Clinical practice points

Neuropathy and bone marrow suppression are rare but potentially serious complications of nitrous oxide use, particularly in at-risk patients

The information about the complications of nitrous oxide comes from case reports only. There are no controlled studies that evaluate the safety of repeated intermittent exposure to nitrous oxide in humans, and no data to guide the appropriate maximum duration or number of times a patient can safely be exposed to nitrous oxide. The suggestions for use of nitrous oxide are extrapolations only from the information above. Consideration should be given to duration of exposure and supplementation with vitamin B_{12}, methionine, and folic or folinic acid

If nitrous oxide is used with other sedative or analgesic agents, appropriate clinical monitoring should be performed

Reproduced with permission from Acute Pain Management: Scientific Evidence ANZCA and FPM (2005)

NMDA receptor antagonist drugs

Tissue damage or inflammation, such as that occurring after surgery or trauma, causes pain stimuli to be carried along peripheral sensory nerves to the spinal cord. Persistent input of pain stimuli from the site of injury leads to changes in the way in which spinal cord neurons process the information received from the periphery.

Repetitive input of painful stimuli can lead to the development of spinal cord neuron hyperexcitability, a process referred to as *central sensitization*. Symptoms of this process include increased sensitivity and an exaggerated response to further pain stimuli (*hyperalgesia*). The increased sensitivity may also extend to stimuli that would not normally be regarded as painful (e.g. touch), but which because of these changes result in the sensation of pain (*allodynia*). Thus, central sensitization leads to alterations in the nature of the pain perceived or increases in its intensity and duration.

Underlying phenomena in the spinal cord include w*ind-up*, where spinal cord neurons show a progressively greater response to repetitive but constant intensity stimuli. This is caused by prolonged glutamate release and its activation of *N*-methyl-D-aspartate (NMDA) receptors in dorsal horn neurons. Other phenomena involved include *long-term potentiation, recruitment* leading to expansion of the receptive fields of these neurons, *afterdischarge* and increased spontaneous neuronal activity. These processes happen in all patients after acute injury. In most patients central sensitization appears to be reversed as the injury heals and acute pain resolves. In some patients, however, the condition becomes chronic (see also Chapter 12). It is also of note that tolerance to opioids may have a pathophysiological basis similar to that of central sensitization.

There is evidence for NMDA receptor involvement in many types of pain: inflammatory, postoperative, neuropathic and ischemic. Drugs that act as antagonists at these receptors may not only prevent the development of wind-up and central sensitization, but may also downregulate hyperexcitability after sensitization has taken place. Therefore, NMDA receptor antagonist drugs show effects that are better described as 'antiallodynic', 'antihyperalgesic' and 'tolerance protective' rather than analgesic.

The use of NMDA receptor antagonist drugs is increasingly common in the management of specific acute and chronic pain states (Box 6.3). In acute pain management, relatively low doses are usually administered as an adjunct to other analgesic interventions. Used in such a way they may improve the quality of pain relief and reduce the amount of opioid needed for analgesia, and may reduce the incidence of some opioid-related side effects. They are particularly useful for the treatment of pain that is poorly responsive to opioids, or in opioid-tolerant patients. They may also have a preventive effect in limiting the progression from acute to chronic pain syndromes (such as post-thoracotomy, post-mastectomy and phantom pain) and have been shown to be effective in the treatment of neuropathic pain (see Chapter 12). Last, but not least, in higher doses

---

Box 6.3

Possible uses for NMDA receptor antagonist drugs

'Low-dose use'

- Prevention (?reversal) of central sensitization and wind-up
- Treatment of poorly opioid-responsive pain
- Management of neuropathic pain
- Management of pain in opioid-tolerant patients

'High-dose use'

- Treatment of acute pain

---

they can be used to treat pain in emergencies, in out-of-hospital settings, in disaster scenarios, during transport and transfer, and for procedures such as dressing changes, while causing no or only minimal respiratory depression.

Ketamine

The most common NMDA receptor antagonist in clinical use is ketamine, a compound that was initially developed as a dissociative anesthetic agent. It is still widely used to provide anesthesia in out-of-hospital settings, in disasters, and in developing countries. It is most commonly available as a racemic mixture of *R* and *S* isomers. The *S* isomer, available in some countries only, is a more potent analgesic, has a shorter duration of action, and is claimed to produce fewer side effects than the racemic mixture. Ketamine acts at a number of receptors, including NMDA and opioid receptors, although interactions at receptors other than the NMDA receptor appear to be of limited clinical importance.

The terminal elimination half-life of racemic ketamine is 2–3 hours. The drug is metabolized by the liver and the metabolites are excreted by the kidney. The primary metabolite, norketamine, is less potent than ketamine, but is also an NMDA receptor antagonist and contributes to its analgesic effect.

Clinical efficacy and use

When used in pain management, ketamine is usually administered by IV or SC routes. There is increasing interest and evidence of efficacy for non-parenteral routes of administration (intranasal, transmucosal, transdermal). The use of higher doses requires familiarity with the drug and its adverse effects, although it is the only anesthetic agent that results in no or only minimal respiratory depression or airway compromise.

In contrast to other anesthetic agents, ketamine can provide excellent analgesia when given in subanesthetic doses. The NMDA receptor and opioid-sparing effects of ketamine may be seen with infusion rates as low as $1 \mu g/kg/min$ (about $100 mg/day$ in an average adult). Some centers use an easy-to-calculate initial infusion rate of $0.1 mg/kg/h$ (i.e. $7 mg/h$ for the average adult) and then adjust the rate according to effect and adverse effects. In the older patient it may be appropriate to start with even lower doses (e.g. $50 mg/day$ or $2 mg/h$) and increase as needed.

It may be useful to give a small loading dose prior to the start of the infusion e.g. $100–200 \mu g/kg$ ($5–15 mg$) in the average adult patient, with the lower doses used in elderly patients. Single bolus doses in this range can also be used to treat pain that has not responded well to large doses of opioid ('*rescue analgesia*'), for example in the recovery room.

The addition of ketamine to opioid analgesic regimens can lead to a reduction in opioid requirements (opioid sparing) and may also reduce the incidence of postoperative nausea and vomiting.

In some centers ketamine is added to the opioid used in patient-controlled analgesia (PCA), so that the patient receives both opioid and ketamine with every demand. However, large variations in opioid requirements mean that patients are likely to receive widely varying doses of ketamine. This could lead to inadequate therapy in some patients and an increased risk of adverse effects in others.

High-dose ketamine also has a role in acute pain management. It can be used to provide analgesia for fracture reductions and other painful procedures, e.g. dressing changes. In these situations, doses can be titrated in $10–20 mg$ steps (or less in the older patient), usually in combination with midazolam to reduce the incidence of psychotomimetic adverse effects and prevent nightmares.

The use of bolus doses of $10 mg$ ketamine with $0.5 mg$ midazolam with a 5-minute lockout via PCA pumps for burns dressings has proved very effective, with a high patient acceptance.

Adverse effects

One of the main problems with ketamine is that it interferes with sensory perception as well as the perception of pain. As a result, its use has been associated with psychotomimetic side effects. With higher doses these effects include dreaming and nightmares (pleasant or unpleasant), hallucinations, and excitation, agitation and delirium. These side effects may be reduced by the concurrent administration of benzodiazepines.

With the lower doses mentioned above adverse effects may still occur (albeit infrequently, i.e. in less than 10% of cases). These effects may include dizziness and feelings of unreality or 'floating'. In such cases co-administration of low-dose benzodiazepines, e.g. midazolam, can reduce these effects, although care should be taken in patients also receiving opioids, as this could increase the risk of respiratory depression.

To a large extent these effects are dose related and are probably negligible at doses of less than $2.5\,\mu g/kg/min$, i.e. less than $200\,mg/day$ in the average adult. In some patients up to $300\,mg/day$ may be used without adverse effect; in older patients it may be appropriate to use lower doses, e.g. 50–$100\,mg/day$.

In the low doses used for pain relief, clinically relevant cardiovascular or respiratory effects have not been reported.

Ketamine is used as a recreational drug, and in some settings administration using a locked infusion pump may be appropriate.

Key points

Evidence level

I Ketamine has an opioid-sparing effect in postoperative pain

I NMDA receptor antagonist drugs may show preventive analgesic effects

II Ketamine improves analgesia in patients with severe pain that is poorly responsive to opioids

IV Ketamine may reduce opioid requirements in opioid-tolerant patients

---

Clinical practice point

Ketamine may be a useful adjunct in conditions of allodynia, hyperalgesia and opioid tolerance

Reproduced with permission from Acute Pain Management: Scientific Evidence ANZCA and FPM (2005)

Dextromethorphan

Dextromethorphan is widely available as an over-the-counter cough suppressant. It is not in common clinical use and has shown disappointing analgesic effects in most clinical trials.

α_2-Adrenergic agonist drugs

α_2 Adrenoreceptors (or α_2 receptors) are located on peripheral sensory nerve terminals and in the spinal cord and brain stem. They have an inhibitory effect on pain transmission and explain the analgesic effects of norepinephrine (noradrenaline) reuptake inhibitors such as tramadol and tricyclic antidepressants. These receptors in the spinal cord are thought to be primarily responsible for the analgesic effects of α_2-adrenergic agonist drugs such as clonidine. These drugs are normally used in combination with other analgesic drugs such as local anesthetics or opioids.

Clonidine

Clonidine is the α_2 agonist most commonly used in clinical practice. It is available in tablet or injectable form, the latter for parenteral injection (IV, SC or IM) or addition to solutions used in regional anesthesia or analgesia (including epidural and intrathecal analgesia). A transdermal patch is also available in some countries. Approximately 50% of clonidine is metabolized in the liver, the remainder being excreted unchanged by the kidney.

Introduced initially as a nasal decongestant and used for years as an antihypertensive, clonidine is also an effective analgesic. By itself it has been used for pain relief after a variety of surgical procedures, although it is normally used in combination with other analgesic drugs. In acute pain management, combination with opioid analgesia can lead to improved pain relief and a reduction in opioid requirements. It can be of particular use in opioid-tolerant and opioid-dependent patients, as it reduces the severity of withdrawal symptoms (see below). Added to solutions used for epidural, intrathecal and other major regional (e.g. brachial or lumbar plexus) anesthesia and analgesia, clonidine has been shown to increase the duration of pain relief. In general, administration by epidural, intrathecal and peripheral nerve routes is more effective than IV or oral administration.

The routine use of clonidine in acute pain management has been limited by side effects, particularly hypotension and sedation. Other possible side effects include bradycardia, dizziness, dry mouth, decreased bowel motility, and diuresis.

Clonidine may be effective in the treatment of neuropathic pain and other forms of chronic and cancer pain. It has also been used in the management of withdrawal from opioids, benzodiazepines and alcohol. Abrupt cessation of clonidine after long-term treatment can itself lead to a withdrawal syndrome, the signs and symptoms of which can include restlessness, headache, nausea, insomnia, rebound hypertension and cardiac arrhythmias.

Dexmedetomidine

Dexmedetomidine is a more specific and shorter-acting α_2 agonist. It is mainly indicated for sedation, particularly in intensive care units. In this setting it has shown an additional benefit in reducing opioid requirements.

Calcitonin

Calcitonin is a peptide hormone that regulates calcium homeostasis. Salmon calcitonin has a higher potency than human calcitonin and is used clinically.

Initial indications were for the treatment of hypercalcemia (e.g. in malignancy with bone metastases) and to increase the calcium content of bones in Paget's disease and osteoporosis. However, when used for these reasons, an analgesic effect was also observed. This was thought to be mediated by modulation of serotoninergic mechanisms, but it may also act as a neurotransmitter in the CNS.

In pain therapy it has proven efficacy in the treatment of acute phantom limb pain and acute pain due to vertebral body fractures, and for the management of chronic pain in complex regional pain syndrome (CRPS) and bone metastases. However, in the latter condition bisphosphonates seem to be more effective.

Although calcitonin is available in some countries for intranasal administration, it is most commonly given by intravenous infusion or, more conveniently, by SC injection. Most reports use daily doses in the range of 100–200 IU of salmon calcitonin for a treatment series of a number of days.

Nausea and vomiting are the most common adverse effects, and premedication with an antiemetic, preferably metoclopramide, can prevent this to a large extent. Flushing and drowsiness are other adverse effects; allergic reactions and hypocalcemia occur rarely, if ever.

Antidepressant drugs

Tricyclic antidepressants (TCAs) are commonly used as first-line agents in the treatment of neuropathic pain and have been shown to be effective in a variety of neuropathic pain states. The analgesic effect of these drugs is distinct from the effect on mood, as pain relief can be obtained in the absence of depression. These drugs may also help 'normalize' sleep patterns. Effects on pain and sleep are likely to be seen at relatively low doses and within a few days of starting treatment, whereas antidepressant effects may require several weeks and higher doses.

Mechanism of action

Tricyclic antidepressants inhibit the reuptake of monoamines into nerve terminals and modulate pain sensation via descending inhibitory pathways in the spinal cord. Classic TCAs (e.g. amitriptyline, imipramine), which inhibit the reuptake of norepinephrine (noradrenaline) and serotonin (5-hydroxytryptamine, 5HT), appear to be the most effective in the treatment of neuropathic pain. Newer antidepressants, such as selective serotonin reuptake inhibitors (SSRIs), which inhibit the reuptake of serotonin only, may have fewer side effects but have not been shown to be as effective in neuropathic pain. The TCAs also block sodium channels and α_2-adrenergic receptors and have NMDA receptor antagonist properties; these actions may contribute to their analgesic effects.

Amitriptyline is the most widely studied TCA of those used in chronic pain states. However, other TCAs, such as its major metabolite nortriptyline, and desipramine and imipramine, also have analgesic activity.

Other newer antidepressants such as venlafaxine, a selective norepinephrine reuptake inhibitor (SNRI), are gaining increasing importance in the treatment of neuropathic pain. Venlafaxine appears to have the same efficacy as TCAs, with a better adverse effect profile. Duloxetine, a selective serotonin and norepinephrine reuptake inhibitors (SSNRI), has been registered in a number of countries for the treatment of diabetic neuropathic pain.

Clinical use

Most of the data currently available on the use of antidepressants relate to the management of chronic pain states such as postherpetic neuralgia or diabetic polyneuropathy; data on the use of these agents in acute neuropathic pain are limited to acute zoster and postsurgical pain, where they may also have some preventive effects. They play no role in the treatment of acute nociceptive pain.

Because tolerance develops to both the anticholinergic and the sedative effects of TCAs, it is preferable to start these drugs at a low, single daily dose and to increase it every few days as necessary. As TCAs may cause drowsiness, especially in the early stages of treatment, doses are best given at night.

Preferred starting doses for amitriptyline are 5–10 mg in patients over 60 and 10–25 mg in those under 60. Doses may be increased by 10 mg or 25 mg (depending on patient age) every 3–5 days if required. A satisfactory response usually occurs at levels between 25 mg and 100 mg. Alternative TCAs include nortriptyline, dothiepin, doxepin, imipramine and desimipramine. Care must be taken if the patient is already taking an SSRI. If TCAs are also needed, doses should be reduced and the patient monitored closely for any side effects.

The use of other antidepressants may best be left in the hands of pain specialists.

Adverse effects

Side effects of TCAs result mainly from their anticholinergic actions. They include dry mouth, increased heart rate, blurred vision, constipation and urinary retention. Narrow-angle glaucoma may be aggravated, and arrhythmias can occur. Impairment of cardiac conduction has been reported (usually of more importance in overdose). These drugs may be contraindicated in patients with pre-existing cardiac conduction abnormalities. Sedation is reasonably common.

Key points

Evidence level

I Tricyclic antidepressants are effective in the treatment of chronic neuropathic pain states, chronic headaches and chronic back pain

I In neuropathic pain, tricyclic antidepressants are more effective than selective serotoninergic reuptake inhibitors

II Antidepressants reduce the incidence of chronic neuropathic pain after acute zoster and breast surgery

Clinical practice points

Based on the experience in chronic neuropathic pain states, it would seem reasonable to use tricyclic antidepressants in the management of acute neuropathic pain

To minimize adverse effects, particularly in elderly people, it is advisable to initiate treatment with low doses

Reproduced with permission from Acute Pain Management: Scientific Evidence ANZCA and FPM (2005)

Elderly patients may be more at risk of postural (orthostatic) hypotension, dysphoria, agitation and confusion. Other more serious side effects are rare but include bone marrow depression, skin rashes and hepatic dysfunction.

Anticonvulsant drugs

Anticonvulsant drugs have been shown to be effective in a variety of neuropathic pain states; again, most data come from studies of chronic neuropathic pain. They are thought to work by several mechanisms – the blockade of voltage-gated sodium channels (e.g. carbamazepine, lamotrigine) or calcium channels (e.g. carbamazepine, valproate, lamotrigine, gabapentin, pregabalin) and enhancement of inhibitory GABAergic neurotransmission (e.g. clonazepam) or inhibition of glutamate release (e.g. carbamazepine, valproate, lamotrigine, gabapentin, pregabalin). They are often used on their own in neuropathic pain, or in combination with TCAs, when these alone have failed to produce adequate analgesia.

Beside the drugs discussed below, other anticonvulsants such as felbamate, tiagabine and vigabatrin may be useful in neuropathic pain.

Gabapentinoids

Gabapentin and pregabalin are two anticonvulsants that have become first-line treatment for neuropathic pain in many centers, partly because of their efficacy but also because the incidence of adverse effects is less than with other anticonvulsants. These drugs have been used successfully in a wide range of neuropathic pain conditions, including spinal cord injury and post-amputation pain. They have also shown opioid-sparing effects when used as components of multimodal postoperative analgesia, and preventive effects for some chronic postsurgical pain conditions.

Their effect is based on binding to the $\alpha_2\delta$ subunit of neuronal calcium channels. Gabapentin, the older of the two substances, relies on an active transport mechanism for uptake and therefore has an unreliable dose–response relationship, making titration over a wide dose range (300–3600 mg daily) necessary. It also commonly requires 8-hourly dosing to be effective. Pregabalin was specifically developed for the treatment of neuropathic pain, has a linear dose–response relationship, and should be taken in twice-daily doses of 75–300 mg.

Adverse effects are usually minor, but include drowsiness and dizziness, disturbance of balance and unexplained peripheral edema.

Clonazepam

Clonazepam is a benzodiazepine anticonvulsant and is the only benzodiazepine that has a role to play in the treatment of neuropathic pain. In doses between 0.5 and 2 mg at night it has good efficacy, with adverse effects being limited to sedation. However, as a benzodiazepine it carries the risk of development of tolerance and dependence.

Lamotrigine

Lamotrigine is a newer anticonvulsant that has shown efficacy in peripheral neuropathies, including HIV neuropathy, and also in central pain conditions such as post-stroke pain. Commonly used doses are in the range of 200–400 mg daily. Adverse effects in these doses are limited primarily to dizziness and somnolence.

Carbamazepine

Carbamazepine is structurally related to imipramine. It is often commenced at low doses (e.g. 50–100 mg orally 12-hourly) and increased after a few days if required and if there are no side effects. The range of doses needed to treat neuropathic pain is unknown, but the effective dose is often less than that necessary for seizure control. Its main indication is trigeminal neuralgia, with only limited data for diabetic neuropathy. In a number of countries oxcarbazepine is available as an alternative and has a better adverse effect profile.

As with most older anticonvulsants, adverse effects are reasonably common. During long-term treatment the most frequently reported side effects are blurred vision, drowsiness, ataxia and vertigo. Other possible adverse effects include nausea and vomiting, blood dyscrasias, hepatic dysfunction, and skin reactions such as rashes and Steven–Johnson syndrome.

Sodium valproate

Sodium valproate may also be useful in the treatment of neuropathic pain. Adverse effects are probably less common than with carbamazepine, but include nausea, rashes, ataxia, hepatic dysfunction and thrombocytopenia.

Key points

Evidence level

I Anticonvulsants are effective in the treatment of chronic neuropathic pain states

I Perioperative gabapentin reduces postoperative pain and opioid requirements

Clinical practice point

Based on the experience in chronic neuropathic pain states, it would seem reasonable to use anticonvulsants in the management of acute neuropathic pain

Reproduced with permission from Acute Pain Management: Scientific Evidence ANZCA and FPM (2005)

Membrane-stabilizing drugs

Membrane-stabilizing drugs are used primarily as antiarrhythmics and are thought to work by blocking sodium channels, thereby stabilizing cell membranes and reducing ectopic discharges; the latter are thought to be a major contributor to neuropathic pain states. Lidocaine is particularly useful in the treatment of acute neuropathic pain states, as it can be administered parenterally and has a fast onset of action.

Lidocaine (lignocaine)

The systemic use of this local anesthetic has been shown to be effective in chronic neuropathic pain, especially that due to peripheral nerve trauma. It is also effective in central pain states, including pain from spinal cord injury. In addition, perioperative lidocaine infusions may be analgesic and opioid sparing.

A single dose of IV lidocaine (1–2 mg/kg as a bolus dose over a few minutes or up to 5 mg/kg as a slow infusion over 30–60 minutes) can be given to treat acute neuropathic pain in an emergency situation or to test the effectiveness of this drug. Analgesia from a single dose may exceed by days or weeks the known pharmacological duration of action of the drug. When pain returns, the single dose may be followed by an IV or subcutaneous infusion (1–2 mg/kg/h). It is assumed that sodium channel blockade leads to the suppression of ectopic impulses generated by damaged nerves; these appear to be blocked at concentrations of local anesthetic that are lower than those normally required to block nerve impulses.

Adverse effects include dizziness, perioral numbness, and less frequently a metallic taste, tremor, dry mouth, insomnia, allergic reactions, and tachycardia. Serious adverse events, such as cardiac arrhythmias and hemodynamic instability, have not been reported in clinical trials of this treatment.

Mexiletine

Mexiletine is an antiarrhythmic drug that is structurally related to lidocaine but can be given orally. Although it was thought to be useful as an oral analog of lidocaine, its efficacy in neuropathic pain is rather limited and not commonly predicted by the response to lidocaine.

Adverse effects include nausea, sedation and tremor. Care should be taken in patients with ischemic heart disease or cardiac arrhythmias; sudden cardiac death has been described in susceptible patients. Use of the medication might require monitoring of ECG (QT-interval measurement) and plasma concentrations.

Key points

Evidence level

I Membrane stabilizers are effective in the treatment of chronic neuropathic pain states, particularly after peripheral nerve trauma

II Perioperative intravenous lidocaine (lignocaine) reduces pain on movement and morphine requirements following major abdominal surgery

---

Clinical practice points

Based on the experience in chronic neuropathic pain states, it would seem reasonable to use membrane stabilizers in the management of acute neuropathic pain

Lidocaine (lignocaine) (IV or SC) may be a useful agent to treat acute neuropathic pain

Reproduced with permission from Acute Pain Management: Scientific Evidence ANZCA and FPM (2005)

References and further reading

Australian and New Zealand College of Anaesthetists, Faculty of Pain Medicine. Acute Pain Management: Scientific Evidence, 2nd edn. Melbourne: Australian and New Zealand College of Anaesthetists, 2005. Also available online at: *http://www.anzca.edu.au/publications/acutepain.htm* and *http://www7.health.gov.au/nhmrc/publications/synopses/cp104syn.htm*

Bell RF, Dahl JB, Moore RA et al. (2006) Perioperative ketamine for acute postoperative pain. Cochrane Database of Systematic Reviews, CD004603.

Dahl V, Raeder JC. (2000) Non-opioid postoperative analgesia. Acta Anaesthesiologica Scandinavica 44: 1191–203.

Cheng HF, Harris RC. (2005) Renal effects of non-steroidal anti-inflammatory drugs and selective cyclooxygenase-2 inhibitors. Current Pharmaceutical Design 11: 1795–804.

Eisenach JC, De Kock M, Klimscha W. (1995) α_2-Aadrenergic agonists for regional anesthesia: a clinical review of clonidine. Anesthesiology 85: 655–74.

Elia N, Tramer MR. (2005) Ketamine and postoperative pain – a quantitative systematic review of randomized trials. Pain 113: 61–70.

Finnerup NB, Otto M, McQuay H et al. (2005) Algorithm for neuropathic pain treatment: an evidence based proposal. Pain 118: 289–305.

Gilron I. (2006) Review article: the role of anticonvulsant drugs in postoperative pain management: a bench-to-bedside perspective. Canadian Journal of Anesthesia 53: 562–71.

Graham GG, Scott KF, Day RO. (2005) Tolerability of paracetamol. Drug Safety 28: 227–40.

Hurley RW, Cohen SP, Williams KA et al. (2006) The analgesic effects of perioperative gabapentin on postoperative pain: a meta-analysis. Regional Anesthesia and Pain Medicine 31: 237–47.

Jensen TS. (2002) Anticonvulsants in neuropathic pain: rationale and clinical evidence. European Journal of Pain 6: 61–8.

Kearney PM, Baigent C, Godwin J et al. (2006) Do selective cyclo-oxygenase-2 inhibitors and traditional non-steroidal anti-inflammatory drugs increase the risk of atherothrombosis? Meta-analysis of randomized trials. British Medical Journal 332: 1302–8.

Khan ZP, Ferguson CN, Jones RM. (1999) Alpha-2 and imidazoline receptor agonists: their pharmacology and therapeutic role. Anaesthesia 54: 146–65.

Marrett E, Kurdi O, Zufferey P et al. (2005) Effects of nonsteroidal anti-inflammatory drugs on patient-controlled analgesia morphine side effects. Meta-analysis of randomized controlled trials. Anesthesiology 102: 1083–5.

Maze M, Fujinaga M. (2000) Recent advances in the actions and toxicity of nitrous oxide. Anaesthesia 55: 311–14.

Nunn JF. (1987) Clinical aspects of the interaction between nitrous oxide and vitamin B_{12}. British Journal of Anaesthesia 59: 3–13.

Remy C, Marrett E, Bonnet F. (2005) Effects of acetaminophen on morphine side-effects and consumption after major surgery: meta-analysis of randomized controlled trials. British Journal of Anesthesia 94: 505–13.

Rømsing J, Møniche S. (2004) A systematic review of COX-2 inhibitors compared with traditional NSAIDs, or different COX-2 inhibitors for post-operative pain. Acta Anaesthesiologia Scandinavica 48: 525–46.

Rosen MA. (2002) Nitrous oxide for relief of labor pain: a systematic review. American Journal of Obstetrics and Gynecology 186: S110–26.

Royal College of Anaesthetists. (1998) Guidelines for the use of non-steroidal anti-inflammatory drugs in the perioperative period. London: Royal College of Anaesthetists.

Rumack BH. (2004) Acetaminophen misconceptions. Hepatology 40: 10–15.

Schmid RL, Sandler AN, Katz J. (1999) Use and efficacy of low-dose ketamine in the management of acute postoperative pain: a review of current techniques and outcomes. Pain 82: 111–25.

Schug SA. (2006) The role of COX-2 inhibitors in the treatment of postoperative pain. Journal of Cardiovascular Pharmacology 47: S82–S86.

Schug SA, Garrett WR, Gillespie G. (2003) Opioid and non-opioid analgesics. Best Practice and Research in Clinical Anaesthesiology 17: 91–110.

Sindrup SH, Otto M, Finnerup NB et al. (2005) Antidepressants in the treatment of neuropathic pain. Basic and Clinical Pharmacology and Toxicology 96: 399–409.

Tremont-Lukats IW, Challapalli V, McNicol ED et al. (2005) Systemic administration of local anesthetics to relieve neuropathic pain: a systematic review and meta-analysis. Anesthesia and Analgesia 101: 1738–49.

Tremont-Lukats IW, Megeff C, Backonja, MM. (2000) Anticonvulsants for neuropathic pain syndromes: mechanisms of action and place in therapy. Drugs 60: 1029–52.

Visser EJ. (2005) A review of calcitonin and its use in the treatment of acute pain. Acute Pain 7: 185–9.

Wiebalck CA, Van Aken H. (1995) Paracetamol and propacetamol for postoperative pain: contrasts to traditional NSAIDs. Baillière's Clinical Anaesthesiology 9: 469–81.

Woolf CJ. (1995) Somatic pain – pathogenesis and prevention. British Journal of Anaesthesia 75: 169–76.

Routes of systemic opioid administration

Chapter contents

The introduction of more sophisticated methods for the administration of opioids, such as patient-controlled and epidural analgesia, has undoubtedly improved the management of acute pain for some patients. However, in most centers the majority of patients will still receive opioid medications using one of the more traditional and conventional methods of administration. Surveys continue to show that these methods frequently result in inadequate analgesia, yet only a few attempts have been made to improve their effectiveness.

Lasagna and Beecher (1954) considered the 'optimal' dose of morphine that should be given by subcutaneous (SC) injection for the relief of postoperative pain. After comparing doses of 10 mg and 15 mg, and because the latter had a higher incidence of side effects, they wrote that 'the optimal dose appears to be 10 mg per 70 kg of body weight'. They correctly defined 'optimal dose' as the dose that would give maximum therapeutic effect with minimum adverse effect. However, they unfortunately also cautioned against flexibility in dosing, because of the risk of 'dangerous' side effects, and against high doses because of the 'known' risk of addiction.

Although teaching has changed over the intervening years, the common lack of flexible dose regimens means that traditional methods of pain relief are still often ineffective. Frequently, these regimens make no allowances for the enormous interpatient variation in opioid requirements (eight- to tenfold) that result from the unpredictable differences in pharmacokinetic factors (how the individual patient handles the drug – i.e. how it is absorbed, distributed, metabolized and excreted) and pharmacodynamic factors (how the individual responds to the drug). The same dose of opioid given to different patients can result in a four- to fivefold difference in peak blood level reached; the peak blood concentration from the same dose of opioid may vary twofold within the same patient; and there is at least a five- to tenfold interpatient variation in the minimum effective analgesic concentration (MEAC). Added to this has been the still-common lack of appropriate education of medical and nursing staff, unfounded fears about the risks of side effects and addiction, and a lack of assessment of pain and the patient's response to treatment – both analgesic effect and side effects.

It is therefore hardly surprising that traditional regimens for pain relief may be less than successful. However, to a large extent this continues to be a consequence of deficiencies in their application rather than limitations associated with the route of administration.

The introduction of education programs for medical and nursing staff, and the use of simple guidelines that include treatment algorithms and regular monitoring of pain and significant adverse effects, can lead to major improvements in pain relief. It is also important, where possible, to allow the patient some input into the size and timing of each dose. 'Patient control' should not be confined to patient-controlled analgesia (PCA) pump systems.

Titration of opioids

The key to making any opioid analgesia more effective for the patient is to individualize treatment regimens. As outlined in Chapter 4, blood levels of an opioid need to reach the MEAC – which varies some four- to fivefold between patients – before any relief of pain is perceived. The only way to achieve good pain relief is therefore to titrate the dose for each patient. This requires the prescription of an appropriate initial dose and dose interval followed by monitoring of the effectiveness of analgesia and of signs that would indicate an excessive dose (see Chapter 3), so that subsequent alterations to doses and frequency of administration can be made. The basic requirements for titration of opioids, regardless of route of administration, are summarized in Box 4.5.

The choice of route for opioid administration will depend on many factors. These include the severity, acuity and type of pain, as well as the characteristics of the chosen drug and technique, such as speed of onset, duration and reliability of effect, cost, and patient acceptability. Relevant patient-dependent factors include their ability to use certain techniques of administration and their acceptance of the chosen route.

Oral route

Unless a patient has severe acute pain, and in the absence of any contraindications, oral administration is the route of choice, as it is for many analgesic agents. It is simple, effective and well tolerated by most patients and can be easily continued in an outpatient setting.

Restrictions on the use of this route include delay in gastric emptying, which is common after surgery and injury, and nausea and vomiting. If emptying is delayed, opioids will not pass through to the small intestine where they are absorbed. If several doses are given before normal gastric motility is re-established, accumulated doses may enter the small intestine at the same time when emptying resumes. Once a postoperative or post-injury patient is able to tolerate reasonable amounts of oral fluids, gastric emptying is returning to normal and there is often no need to continue administration of parenteral opioids.

Larger doses are required when opioids are given orally than with parenteral administration (see Chapter 4). This is because of the first-pass effect: that is, the proportion of an orally administered drug that is metabolized by the liver and/or gut wall after absorption from the gastrointestinal tract determines the amount of unchanged drug that reaches the systemic circulation. The equianalgesic doses of oral and parenteral opioids are listed in Box 4.2, which includes tramadol (also discussed in this chapter). Although not strictly an opioid it is often used instead of, or in combination with, an opioid.

Immediate-release or controlled-release formulations

The rate of absorption of orally administered opioids will depend also on the formulation of the drug (e.g. tablet, liquid, or controlled-release). Controlled-release (CR) preparations (also referred to as slow- or extended-release preparations) of opioids such as morphine, oxycodone, hydromorphone and tramadol are commonly used in the treatment of chronic and cancer pain and usually only need to be given once or twice a day on a time-contingent basis and not PRN (*pro re nata*, meaning 'according to circumstances' or 'as the situation requires'). However, the slower onset (often 3–4 hours or more to peak effect) and the longer duration of action of CR formulations make short-term adjustments and rapid titration of the drug impossible. These preparations are therefore unsuitable for the treatment of acute pain, at least in the early stages.

Although methadone has a relatively quick onset of action, its long half-life makes it more difficult to titrate rapidly without risking accumulation of the drug, so it is unsuitable for the routine management of acute pain.

Immediate-release (IR) preparations are preferred for the early management of acute pain using oral opioids. In most cases analgesia will be obtained within 45–60 minutes, hence titration to effect will be easier than with a CR preparation. Such a titration process is often used to establish the appropriate dose of CR opioid, if this is required in the long term.

When patients with chronic or cancer pain are prescribed a CR opioid they are also often ordered an IR opioid for 'breakthrough' analgesia. The amount of IR opioid required can be used as a guide to altering the dose of CR drug. The IR opioid can be given when needed (up to 1-hourly PRN if staffing and monitoring permit; often ordered 2–4-hourly PRN) so that the total amount the patient needs can be rapidly gauged. IR opioids are usually ordered for breakthrough pain in doses of about one-sixth to one-tenth of the total daily CR dose.

Example

A 48-year-old patient with metastatic breast cancer has been prescribed 30 mg CR morphine 12-hourly for pain but says that the pain relief is inadequate. She has also been ordered 3–5 mg morphine syrup 2-hourly PRN:

> She required 8 doses of 5 mg of morphine syrup in 24 hours = 40 mg = 20 mg 12-hourly
>
> Therefore CR morphine could be increased to 50 mg 12-hourly
>
> Breakthrough doses of morphine syrup could be increased to 10–15 mg

A similar method would be used to assess CR oxycodone or hydromorphone doses.

Titration of oral opioids

Dose range

Doses of oral opioid should be based on the age of the patient. If they have been receiving parenteral opioids, particularly via PCA, the parenteral opioid requirement can be used as a guide to the oral dose that is likely to be needed. If a dose – especially one based on prior parenteral requirements – appears to have no effect, a delay in gastric emptying should be suspected and consideration given to returning to parenteral administration.

Oxycodone and codeine are two opioids commonly given orally for the treatment of acute pain. Oxycodone is often classed as a 'weak' opioid, but it is not. The amount that can be given orally is limited only by the number of tablets a patient can reasonably be expected to swallow at one time. If formulations are used where oxycodone is combined with paracetamol (acetaminophen) or aspirin, the limits placed on the doses of these drugs will limit the total amount of oxycodone that can be given in one day. Similarly, oral codeine is commonly administered in a tablet form that combines it with paracetamol, and therefore the amount of codeine that can be given is limited. For these reasons it is more appropriate to provide oral background analgesia with regular paracetamol, and add on-demand doses of an oral opioid such as oxycodone in an immediate-release preparation, than to use combination preparations.

Dose interval

The aims of a dose interval are to allow the previous dose to exert its effect before an additional dose is given and, to a lesser extent, to provide an indication of how long the effect of a single dose might be expected to last. Oral opioids can be ordered as PRN or fixed-interval doses.

Prescriptions of opioids PRN have been the mainstay of acute pain management (albeit often inadequate) for many years. There are both drawbacks and advantages to the PRN system. It should mean that opioid is given when the patient needs it, but there are frequently long delays between the return of discomfort and the actual administration of more opioid. For a variety of reasons a patient may be reluctant to request another dose, at least until the pain is severe. In addition, there are the inevitable delays that follow such a request in many hospitals, as opioids are kept in locked cupboards and extra nurses may be required to check the drug and dose before it is given. Following administration there is yet another delay while the drug takes effect. Unless the patient is offered pain relief frequently, or asks for and is given another dose as soon as the pain starts to become uncomfortable, the PRN system will fail.

The main advantage of a PRN regimen is that, titrated properly, it can provide the flexibility needed to cover the changes in pain stimulus that occur within each patient with acute pain. With these regimens, a dose interval really only has to ensure that a dose of opioid has had its maximum effect before another is given. This will be the time taken for the drug to be absorbed and reach a peak blood concentration plus the time taken to exert its maximum effect on the central nervous system. In most patients this would occur within an hour of oral administration. Therefore, if a patient is in pain, there is no need to wait 4 hours before giving the next dose. A reasonable dose interval that allows for both safety and flexibility would be 1–2 hours. This does not mean that the drug has to be given every 1 or 2 hours but that it can be given if needed.

Oral opioids can also be given at fixed intervals. One reason for this approach being less popular than PRN regimens may be that opioid requirements vary enormously between patients and can be difficult to predict. In addition, especially after major injury or surgery, the level of pain can fluctuate markedly within each patient according to different stimuli (physiotherapy or dressing changes, for example) as well as decrease a little each day. Fixed-interval dosing may not allow adequate flexibility and coverage of these episodes of 'incident' pain, or allow for the progressive reduction in dose requirements that will occur as the patient recovers. If fixed-interval regimens are used a range of doses should be available and the interval may need to be less than the traditional 4 hours. Additional PRN opioid orders may also be needed for breakthrough pain.

Knowledge of a patient's prior opioid requirements (e.g. if they are switching from PCA to oral analgesia) makes calculating oral doses much easier as it gives a good guide to their likely 24-hour oral requirements. Ideally, the patient should be allowed to choose the dose of opioid from the range ordered based on the effect of previous doses (see Chapter 8). The range ordered needs to take into account the fact that the intensity of postoperative pain will decrease rapidly over the first few days in most patients.

Monitoring

As outlined in Chapter 3, monitoring of pain scores, sedation scores and respiratory rates will give an indication of 'how much is enough' and 'how much is too much' opioid. These should be monitored on a regular basis and include an assessment of the patient about an hour after the dose was given, that is, at the time when the peak effect of the drug is likely to occur. Subsequent doses can be adjusted according to the patient's pain and sedation scores.

As with all opioids the aim is to make the patient comfortable while keeping the sedation score less than 2 (see Box 4.5).

Selection of subsequent doses

Although the dose range ordered and the initial dose given should be based on the age of the patient, subsequent doses need to be titrated to suit the individual. All too often subsequent doses are chosen because 'that was the dose given before', and not on the basis of patient assessment. A protocol similar to that suggested below for IM (intramuscular) and SC (subcutaneous) opioids can be used for oral opioid administration, after appropriate alterations have been made to the doses used.

An example protocol for titration of oral immediate-release oxycodone, including age-based doses and monitoring requirements, is outlined in Box 7.1.

Tramadol can also be used. Immediate-release oral tramadol can be ordered as 'tramadol 50–100 mg PRN 1-hourly PRN to a maximum 24-hour dose of 1000 mg'.

Where possible, patients should be allowed some input into the size and timing of subsequent doses. They can be instructed to ask for a larger subsequent dose if analgesia was inadequate, or a smaller dose if they felt sleepy or nauseated.

Intramuscular and subcutaneous routes

Although morphine was first given by SC injection, the IM route has become more common, possibly in the (somewhat mistaken) belief that absorption is slower from subcutaneous sites.

Traditionally, IM opioids have been ordered 4-hourly PRN. A reluctance to give opioids more frequently than this has a major role in the lack of effectiveness of IM regimens. Even if pain returns before the end of this period (which is not uncommon), patients are often made to wait until the 4 hours has elapsed before they are 'allowed' another injection.

Figure 7.1 is a hypothetical representation of what could happen to the blood concentrations of a typical opioid with a half-life of about 3 hours (e.g. morphine) if a fixed IM dose is repeated at 4-hourly intervals.

After absorption from the injection site the first dose may result in a blood level that only just enters the 'analgesic corridor' (range of therapeutic blood concentrations) for that patient, leading to very little if any pain relief. The second two doses may result in higher blood levels and better pain relief for longer periods. Fourth and subsequent doses may increase blood concentrations to a level that, as well as giving pain relief, starts to produce side effects.

Two things are obvious from Figure 7.1:

- The amount of opioid required to make a patient comfortable in the first instance may not be the same as that required to maintain comfort.
- Although peaks and troughs in the blood levels of opioid are an inevitable consequence of this type of regimen, the aim of treatment should be to reduce the extent of this variation so that the peaks and troughs

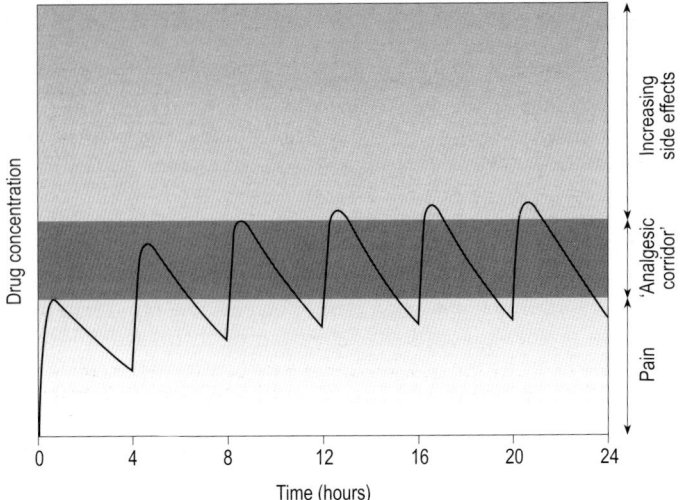

Figure 7.1   Intermittent intramuscular opioid analgesia.

occur predominantly within the 'analgesic corridor'. For example, giving a little less opioid more often can result in the same overall daily dose but less variability in blood concentrations between doses.

The SC route is often used for opioid administration in the treatment of cancer pain and has now become increasingly popular in the management of acute pain. Morphine is the drug most commonly used for intermittent SC injection. The rate of uptake of morphine into the circulation after injection into subcutaneous tissue is similar to that following an IM injection.

An indwelling narrow-gauge 'butterfly' needle or small IV cannula is inserted into subcutaneous tissue – for ease of access often just below the clavicle – and covered with a transparent dressing. To ensure that the needle is placed correctly and not too superficially, a generous fold of skin and subcutaneous tissue should be held in one hand and the needle or cannula inserted at the base of this fold (at an angle of 30–45° to the patient) with the other. Injections can be administered through a cap or one-way valve on the indwelling needle. Advantages of using this route over the IM route include improved patient comfort, as the number of skin punctures is reduced, and a reduced risk of needlestick injury – once the indwelling needle or cannula is in place, all other needles can be avoided.

If the injection through the indwelling needle is painful it may be that the rate of injection is too rapid (each dose needs to be given over 1–2 minutes) or that the needle has been inserted too superficially. The insertion

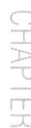

Box 7.1

Royal Adelaide Hospital Guidelines
DOSAGE GUIDELINES FOR INTERMITTENT IMMEDIATE-RELEASE ORAL OXYCODONE ADMINISTRATION
For acute pain management

RAH Drug Committee
Revised June 2004

- Recommended opioid doses are based on average analgesic requirements of opioid-naive patients following moderate to major surgery

- Avoid co-administration of sedatives with opioids where possible

- Avoid co-administration of other opioids - ensure 1 hour has lapsed since the last dose when changing to a different immediate-release opioid.

- Consideration should be given to dosage amendment in differing clinical situations.

- Dose requirements of opioids for analgesia for patients on long term opioid therapy may be higher.

- The best clinical predictor of opioid dose is patient age[1]

- Slow-release oxycodone (Oxycontin) is not recommended for management of acute pain. At the RAH, patients can only be commenced on Oxycontin by the Pain Management, Palliative Care or Cancer Services

[1] Macintyre PE, Jarvis DA. Age is the best predictor of postoperative morphine requirements. Pain 64(2): 357-64 1996

Table: Initial immediate - release oral Oxycodone orders

Age (Years)	Oxycodone Dose range (mg)	
< 15	*	
15 - 39	15 - 25	
40 - 59	10 - 20	
60 - 69	5 - 15	
70 - 85	5 - 10	
> 85	2.5 - 5	

Please direct any queries to:
- Acute Pain Service OR
- Medicines Information Centre Pharmacy Department Phone 25546

* Contact WCH Drug Information Centre or WCH Department of Anaesthesia for advice on opioid doses for children <15 years

- Order recommended dose of opioid 2 hourly prn.
- Suggest start in middle of dose range.
- Upper limit of dose range can be increased if analgesia is inadequate, and if sedation score is less than 2 and respiratory rate greater than 8/min.

Use of Oxycodone as a discharge medication

- Oxycodone is not recommended for routine prescription on discharge
- If it is to be prescribed, both the patient and the patient's general practitioner should be informed that it is recommended that it be used only for a maximum of a week after discharge and in decreasing daily doses. Re-prescription is not recommended. If the patient's pain persists they should be reviewed.

MONITORING OF THERAPY IS ESSENTIAL
For monitoring requirements, refer to RAH Guidelines for Intermittent Oral Oxycodene Administration

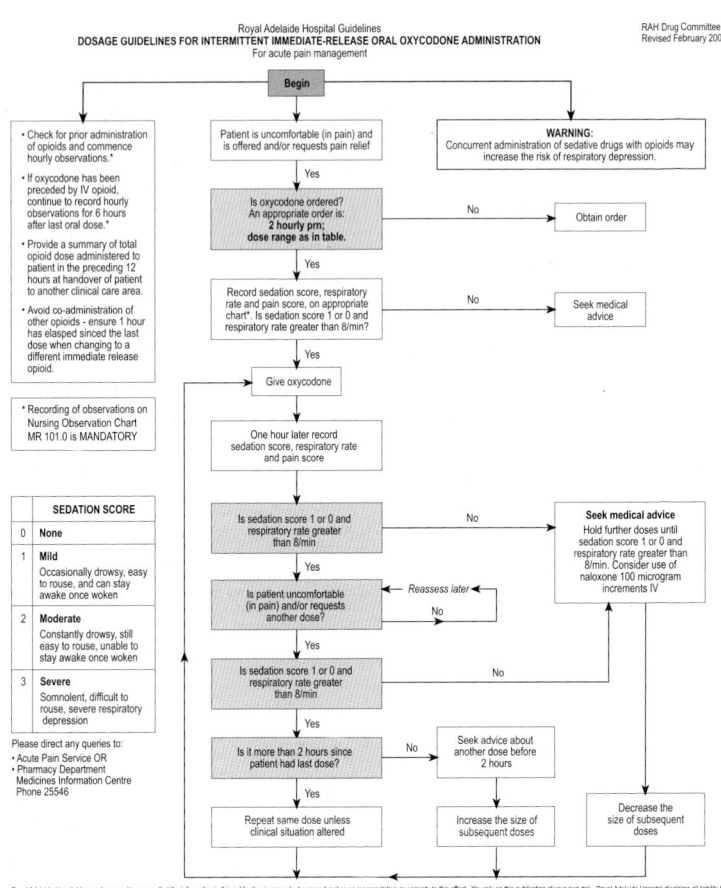

Royal Adelaide Hospital Guidelines
DOSAGE GUIDELINES FOR INTERMITTENT IMMEDIATE-RELEASE ORAL OXYCODONE ADMINISTRATION
For acute pain management

RAH Drug Committee
Revised February 2004

Begin

- Check for prior administration of opioids and commence hourly observations.*
- If oxycodone has been preceded by IV opioid, continue to record hourly observations for 6 hours after last oral dose.*
- Provide a summary of total opioid dose administered to patient in the preceding 12 hours at handover of patient to another clinical care area.
- Avoid co-administration of other opioids - ensure 1 hour has elapsed sinced the last dose when changing to a different immediate release opioid.

* Recording of observations on Nursing Observation Chart MR 101.0 is MANDATORY

SEDATION SCORE	
0	**None**
1	**Mild** Occasionally drowsy, easy to rouse, and can stay awake once woken
2	**Moderate** Constantly drowsy, still easy to rouse, unable to stay awake once woken
3	**Severe** Somnolent, difficult to rouse, severe respiratory depression

Please direct any queries to:
- Acute Pain Service OR
- Pharmacy Department Medicines Information Centre Phone 25546

Patient is uncomfortable (in pain) and is offered and/or requests pain relief
→ Yes

Is oxycodone ordered? An appropriate order is: **2 hourly prn; dose range as in table.** — No → Obtain order
→ Yes

Record sedation score, respiratory rate and pain score, on appropriate chart*. Is sedation score 1 or 0 and respiratory rate greater than 8/min? — No → Seek medical advice
→ Yes

Give oxycodone

One hour later record sedation score, respiratory rate and pain score

Is sedation score 1 or 0 and respiratory rate greater than 8/min — No → **Seek medical advice** Hold further doses until sedation score 1 or 0 and respiratory rate greater than 8/min. Consider use of naloxone 100 microgram increments IV
→ Yes

Is patient uncomfortable (in pain) and/or requests another dose? ← Reassess later — No →
→ Yes

Is sedation score 1 or 0 and respiratory rate greater than 8/min — No →
→ Yes

Is it more than 2 hours since patient had last dose? — No → Seek advice about another dose before 2 hours
→ Yes

Repeat same dose unless clinical situation altered | Increase the size of subsequent doses | Decrease the size of subsequent doses

WARNING: Concurrent administration of sedative drugs with opioids may increase the risk of respiratory depression.

Royal Adelaide Hospital has endeavoured to ensure that the information in this publication is accurate, however it makes no representation or warranty to this effect. You rely on this publication at your own risk. Royal Adelaide Hospital disclaims all liability for any claims, losses, damages, costs and expenses suffered or incurred as a result of reliance on this publication. As the information in this publication is subject to review, please contact a medical or health professional before using this publication.

site should be changed if pain on injection persists, or if any redness or swelling develops at the site. Normally the indwelling needle will only need to be replaced every 3–4 days, although some institutions may require all indwelling cannulae to be changed more frequently.

Subcutaneous opioids should be given in solutions concentrated enough to avoid the need for large volumes, as this can be another source of tissue irritation and pain.

Titration of intermittent IM or SC opioids

The principles of titration for IM and SC opioids are very similar to those for oral opioids.

Dose range

As for any route, an age-related range of doses should be prescribed initially. A guide to total daily morphine doses can be obtained from Figure 4.1. Division of these 24-hour doses by 8 gives a reasonable indication of a value for the middle of an appropriate dose range for patients of a particular age. Although division by 8 estimates a 3-hourly dose, it is reasonable to add additional flexibility by ordering the range of doses more frequently (see below).

Suggestions for initial dose ranges (based on Figure 4.1) are listed in Box 7.2. Note that these values were obtained from opioid-naive patients using morphine by PCA after major surgery. Dose requirements may be lower following less major surgery, or higher for patients with a history of prior opioid use. Variations may also occur in different patient populations.

Staff are often tempted to start at the lower limit of any prescribed range, but these ranges should allow them to reduce as well as increase subsequent doses as necessary. Unless there is a contraindication (e.g. the patient has severe pain or is a little sleepy), and provided the range ordered is appropriate, it is reasonable to start in the middle of the range in most cases.

Dose interval

As with oral regimens, IM and SC opioids can be ordered as PRN or fixed-interval doses, and the comments made above relating to oral opioid analgesia apply. A PRN regimen is commonly used in the acute setting because of the rapidly changing nature of acute pain, but analgesic efficacy will be very dependent on the patient getting the appropriate dose truly when needed. As most of the effect of an IM or SC opioid dose will be seen well within 45–60 minutes, dose intervals of just 1 hour are possible, provided there is proper ongoing monitoring and assessment of the patient. A delay in absorption may be seen where there is poor perfusion, such as in hypovolemic or hypothermic states. This may lead to late onset of analgesia and late absorption of the drug when perfusion is restored. In such situations intravenous (IV) administration is preferred.

Monitoring and selection of subsequent doses

Pain scores, sedation scores and respiratory rate should be monitored on a regular basis. For intermittent IM and SC regimens it would be reasonable to record these values when an injection is given (assuming it is given truly 'on demand') and 1 hour later, when the full effect of the injection can be seen.

Box 7.2

Royal Adelaide Hospital Guidelines
DOSAGE GUIDELINES FOR INTERMITTENT SUBCUTANEOUS OPIOID ADMINISTRATION
For acute pain management

RAH Drug Committee
Revised June 2004

- Subcutaneous, rather than intramuscular, administration is recommended
- For intermittent administration of intravenous opioids refer to appropriate RAH guidelines

- Recommended opioid doses are based on average analgesic requirements of opioid-naive patients following moderate to major surgery

- Avoid co-administration of sedatives with opioids where possible

- Avoid co-administration of other opioids - ensure 1 hour has lapsed since the last dose when changing to a different immediate-release opioid.

- Consideration should be given to dosage amendment in differing clinical situations.

- Dose requirements of opioids for analgesia for patients on long term opioid therapy may be higher.

- The best clinical predictor of opioid dose is patient age[1]

[1] Macintyre PE, Jarvis DA. Age is the best predictor of postoperative morphine requirements. Pain 64(2): 357-64 1996

Table: Initial Opioid orders		
Age (Years)	**Morphine Dose range (mg)**	**Hydromorphone Dose range (mg)**
<15	*	*
15 - 39	7.5 - 12.5	1.5 - 2.5
40 - 59	5.0 - 10.0	1.0 - 2.0
60 - 69	2.5 - 7.5	0.5 - 1.5
70 - 85	2.5 - 5.0	0.5 - 1.0
> 85	2.0 - 3.0	0.4 - 0.6

Please direct any queries to:
- Acute Pain Service OR
- Medicines Information Centre Pharmacy Department Phone 25546

* Contact WCH Drug Information Centre or WCH Department of Anaesthesia for advice on opioid doses for children <15 years

- Order recommended dose of opioid 2 hourly prn.
- Suggest start in middle of dose range.
- Upper limit of dose range can be increased if analgesia is inadequate, and if sedation score is less than 2 and respiratory rate greater than 8/min.

Use of Hydromorphone

- Hydromorphone is second-line opioid
  Note that hydromorphone is approximately five times as potent as morphine
  SC hydromorphone 1.3mg–2mg is equivalent in efficacy and potential adverse effects to SC morphine 10mg

MONITORING OF THERAPY IS ESSENTIAL
For monitoring requirements, refer to RAH Guidelines for Intermittent Subcutaneous Opioid Administration

An example protocol for titration of intermittent IM or SC opioids, including age-based doses and monitoring requirements, is outlined in Box 7.2. Similar algorithms have been shown to lead to significant improvements in pain relief.

Where possible, patients should be allowed some input into the size and timing of subsequent doses. They can be instructed to ask for a

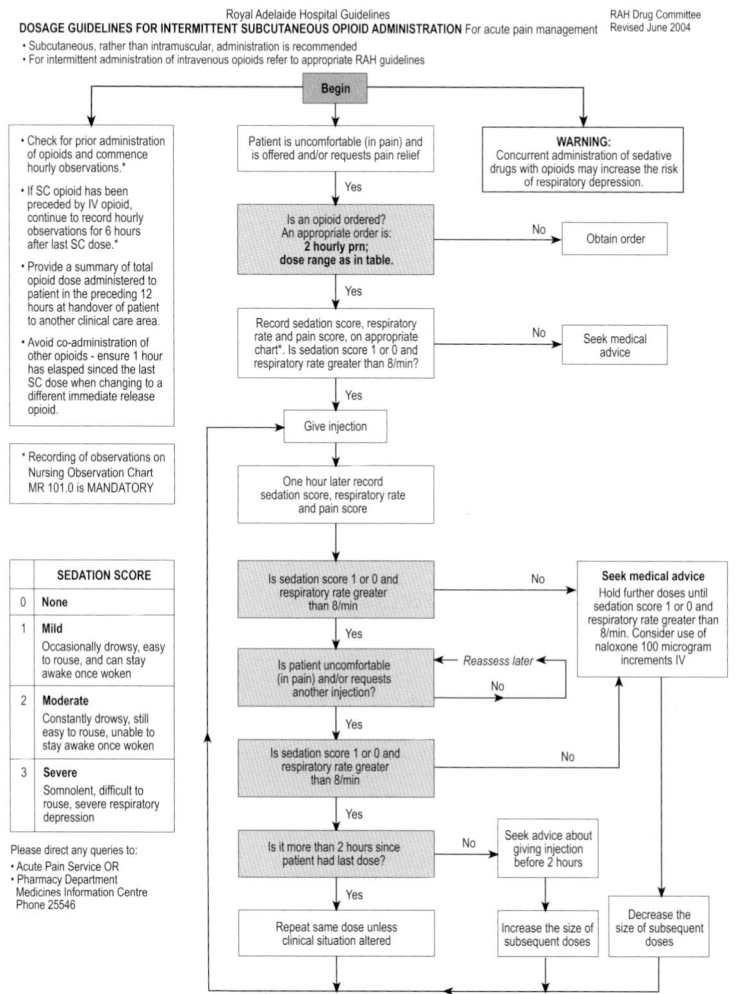

Royal Adelaide Hospital Guidelines
DOSAGE GUIDELINES FOR INTERMITTENT SUBCUTANEOUS OPIOID ADMINISTRATION For acute pain management
RAH Drug Committee
Revised June 2004
• Subcutaneous, rather than intramuscular, administration is recommended
• For intermittent administration of intravenous opioids refer to appropriate RAH guidelines

Begin

• Check for prior administration of opioids and commence hourly observations.*

• If SC opioid has been preceded by IV opioid, continue to record hourly observations for 6 hours after last SC dose.*

• Provide a summary of total opioid dose administered to patient in the preceding 12 hours at handover of patient to another clinical care area.

• Avoid co-administration of other opioids - ensure 1 hour has elapsed sinced the last SC dose when changing to a different immediate release opioid.

* Recording of observations on Nursing Observation Chart MR 101.0 is MANDATORY

Patient is uncomfortable (in pain) and is offered and/or requests pain relief

WARNING:
Concurrent administration of sedative drugs with opioids may increase the risk of respiratory depression.

Yes

Is an opioid ordered? An appropriate order is: **2 hourly prn; dose range as in table.** — No → Obtain order

Yes

Record sedation score, respiratory rate and pain score, on appropriate chart*. Is sedation score 1 or 0 and respiratory rate greater than 8/min? — No → Seek medical advice

Yes

Give injection

One hour later record sedation score, respiratory rate and pain score

Is sedation score 1 or 0 and respiratory rate greater than 8/min — No → **Seek medical advice**
Hold further doses until sedation score 1 or 0 and respiratory rate greater than 8/min. Consider use of naloxone 100 microgram increments IV

Yes

Is patient uncomfortable (in pain) and/or requests another injection? ← Reassess later — No

Yes

Is sedation score 1 or 0 and respiratory rate greater than 8/min — No

Yes

Is it more than 2 hours since patient had last dose? — No → Seek advice about giving injection before 2 hours

Yes

Repeat same dose unless clinical situation altered

Increase the size of subsequent doses

Decrease the size of subsequent doses

	SEDATION SCORE
0	**None**
1	**Mild** Occasionally drowsy, easy to rouse, and can stay awake once woken
2	**Moderate** Constantly drowsy, still easy to rouse, unable to stay awake once woken
3	**Severe** Somnolent, difficult to rouse, severe respiratory depression

Please direct any queries to:
• Acute Pain Service OR
• Pharmacy Department Medicines Information Centre Phone 25546

Royal Adelaide Hospital has endeavoured to ensure that the information in this publication is accurate, however it makes no representation or warrenty to this effect. You rely on this publication at your own risk. Royal Adelaide Hospital disclaims all liability for any claims, losses, damages, costs and expenses suffered or incurred as a result of reliance of this publication. As the information in this publication is subject t review, please contact a medical or health professional before using this publication.

larger subsequent dose if analgesia was inadequate, or a smaller dose if they felt sleepy or nauseated.

Intravenous route

Many books and guidelines still suggest that IV opioids should be given in doses similar to those administered by IM injection and at similar intervals. Figure 7.2 is a hypothetical representation of what might happen to opioid blood levels if the *same dose* as administered by IM injection in Figure 7.1 were given by IV injection every 4 hours. This regimen would result in large variations in blood concentrations of the drug. It is therefore not a particularly effective – and, more importantly, a potentially unsafe – way of administering opioids. If sustained pain relief is to be obtained without side effects, much smaller doses must be given intravenously much more often.

The smaller the dose and the more often it can be administered, the less variability there will be in the blood levels of the drug and the easier it will be to titrate the drug to suit each patient and differing pain stimuli. This is the rationale behind PCA and one of the reasons why it has been so effective. However, it would be a major logistical and staffing problem if intermittent IV doses of opioid had to be given by nursing staff to large numbers of patients, so this method is not recommended for

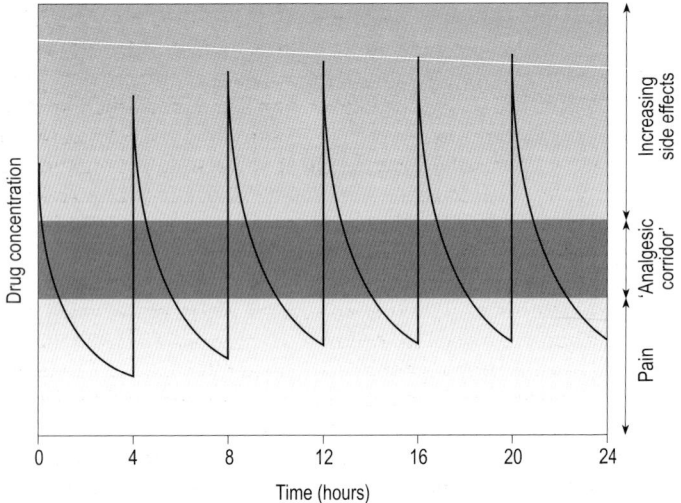

Figure 7.2 Intermittent intravenous opioid analgesia.

routine maintenance of pain relief in general wards. This technique is, however, the best way to obtain rapid analgesia and should be used to:

- obtain initial pain relief (e.g. immediately after an operation), i.e. 'load' the patient so that blood levels rapidly reach the MEAC for that patient;
- provide analgesia for patients who are hypovolemic or hypotensive, when uptake of drug from muscle or subcutaneous tissue is poor;
- cover episodes of 'incident pain' (e.g. dressing changes, physiotherapy) or inadequate analgesia.

In an attempt to avoid the 'peaks and troughs' in blood concentration associated with intermittent administration, continuous IV infusions of opioid are sometimes used in the management of acute pain. Although it may be possible to maintain reasonably constant blood levels using this technique, it is difficult to predict what the level will need to be for a particular patient, or what dose is needed to achieve it. Also, acute pain is not constant and the amount of opioid required by a patient will vary in response to different pain stimuli. For the reasons outlined below, alterations of infusion rate alone will often mean there is a considerable delay in matching the amount of opioid delivered to the amount actually needed. There are also possible risks from blood levels of the drug that may continue to rise after analgesia has been obtained.

If an infusion of any drug is ordered at a fixed rate, it takes five half-lives of the drug to reach 95% of final steady-state concentration. The half-life of morphine is 2–3 hours, so it may take up to 15 hours for blood levels to reach a plateau at this steady-state concentration. It is this plateau that needs to be in the 'analgesic corridor'.

It can be seen from the hypothetical representation in Figure 7.3 of a continuous infusion of an opioid with a half-life of 3 hours (e.g. morphine) that analgesia has been obtained within 3 hours of starting the infusion. If this infusion continues at the same rate, the blood concentration will continue to rise for some hours, and side effects (including respiratory depression) may result. It will also take hours for each alteration made to the infusion rate to have its full effect, i.e. to reach the new steady-state concentration – a fact often not recognized by staff, who may change the rates as often as every 30 minutes.

A patient who becomes sedated while using PCA (PCA mode only) will not press the demand button and further doses of drug will not be delivered. Equipment used for continuous infusions of opioid will continue to deliver the drug regardless of whether the patient is sedated or not. For this reason continuous IV infusions are probably the *least safe* way to administer opioids in a general ward.

As tramadol is less likely to cause respiratory depression than equianalgesic doses of conventional opioids, it may be a safer option for a continuous infusion in the ward setting.

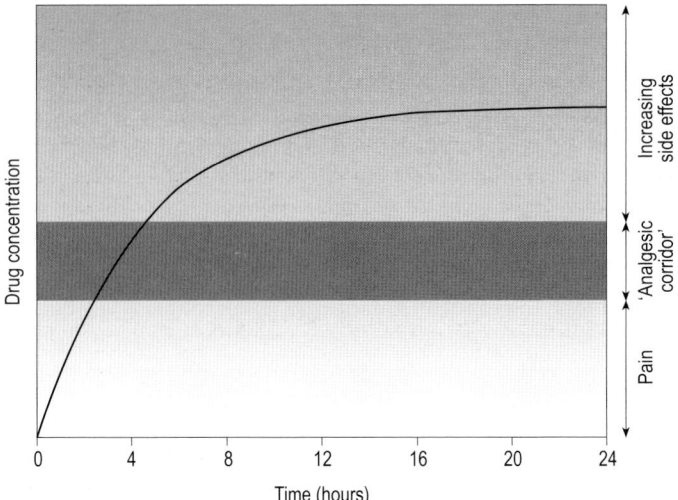

Figure 7.3 Continuous intravenous opioid infusions.

Titration of intermittent IV opioids

Dose range

As before, dose ranges should be based on the age of the patient. Suggested doses for morphine and fentanyl are listed in Box 7.3.

Dose interval

It may take 15 minutes or more for a less lipid-soluble drug such as morphine to exert its maximum effect on the central nervous system after IV administration. However, this is too long if analgesia is to be obtained rapidly. A reasonable balance between absolute safety (ensuring that one dose has had its peak effect before another is given) and efficacy is to use a dose interval of 3–5 minutes. This has proved safe and effective, as long as staff monitor the patient carefully and are aware that this interval may not represent the true time to peak effect.

Monitoring and selection of subsequent doses

A protocol that has been widely used for the administration of intermittent IV bolus doses of opioid is reproduced in Box 7.3. It is managed by nursing staff, usually in the post-anesthesia recovery area, or other specialized areas such as the burns unit. There is no limit to the total amount of opioid that can be given. While this protocol is in use, and for 15 minutes after its cessation, a nurse should remain close to the patient.

Subsequent analgesic regimens

Patients given intermittent IV opioids will normally be changed to an alternative analgesic regimen once they are comfortable. If PCA is to be used it can be started immediately. If IM or SC opioids are ordered, a dose should be given at the earliest sign of discomfort.

Titration of continuous IV opioid infusions

Dose range

In view of the variable time taken from the start of a continuous infusion to the onset of pain relief, analgesia will be obtained more rapidly if IV bolus doses (as in Box 7.3) are administered to 'load' the patient in the first instance, and the infusion is commenced once they are comfortable. It has been said that the rate of the infusion can then be based on this loading dose, half the loading dose being required during each elimination

---

Box 7.3

Dilution method for 10 ml syringe
Draw up **10 mg morphine** or **200 micrograms fentanyl** and make up to 10 ml with sodium chloride 0.9%

Dilution method for 20 ml syringe
Draw up **20 mg morphine** or **400 micrograms fentanyl** and make up to 20 ml with sodium chloride 0.9%

	SEDATION SCORE
0	**None**
1	**Mild** Occasionally drowsy, easy to rouse, and can stay awake once woken
2	**Moderate** Constantly drowsy, still easy to rouse, unable to stay awake once woken
3	**Severe** Somnolent, difficult to rouse, severe respiratory depression

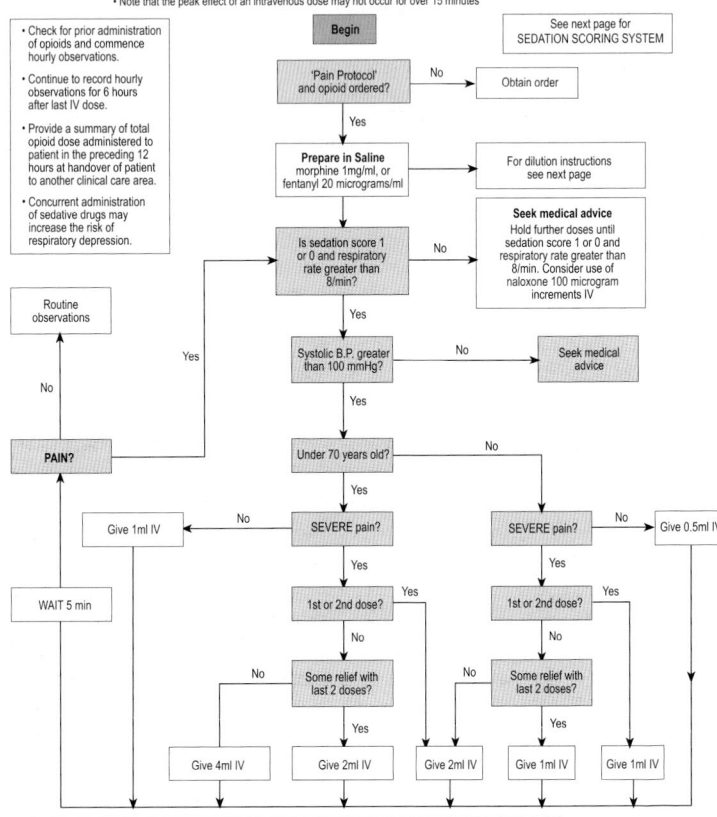

Royal Adelaide Hospital Guidelines
DOSAGE GUIDELINES FOR INTERMITTENT INTRAVENOUS OPIOID ADMINISTRATION For acute pain management

Please direct any queries to Acute Pain Service

USE OF THESE GUIDELINES IS RESTRICTED TO RECOVERY WARDS, EMERGENCY DEPARTMENT, BURNS UNIT, P4IC, P4SD, B4, D6
- Only to be used by staff who have been instructed in this technique
- NOT appropriate for routine maintenance of analgesia in general wards
- Note that the peak effect of an intravenous dose may not occur for over 15 minutes

- Check for prior administration of opioids and commence hourly observations.
- Continue to record hourly observations for 6 hours after last IV dose.
- Provide a summary of total opioid dose administered to patient in the preceding 12 hours at handover of patient to another clinical care area.
- Concurrent administration of sedative drugs may increase the risk of respiratory depression.

See next page for SEDATION SCORING SYSTEM

Begin

'Pain Protocol' and opioid ordered? — No → Obtain order
Yes

Prepare in Saline morphine 1mg/ml, or fentanyl 20 micrograms/ml → For dilution instructions see next page

Is sedation score 1 or 0 and respiratory rate greater than 8/min? — No → **Seek medical advice** Hold further doses until sedation score 1 or 0 and respiratory rate greater than 8/min. Consider use of naloxone 100 microgram increments IV
Yes

Routine observations

Systolic B.P. greater than 100 mmHg? — No → Seek medical advice
Yes

No

PAIN?

Under 70 years old? — No
Yes

Give 1ml IV ← No — SEVERE pain?   SEVERE pain? — No → Give 0.5ml IV
Yes   Yes

WAIT 5 min

1st or 2nd dose? — Yes   1st or 2nd dose? — Yes
No   No

Some relief with last 2 doses? — No   Some relief with last 2 doses? — No → Give 2ml IV
Yes   Yes

Give 4ml IV   Give 2ml IV   Give 2ml IV   Give 1ml IV   Give 1ml IV

If within an hour, a patient under 70 years of age requires more than 20 mg morphine (400 micrograms fentanyl), or a patient over 70 years of age more than 10 mg morphine (or 200 micrograms fentanyl), seek medical advice.

Royal Adelaide Hospital has endeavoured to ensure that the information in this publication is accurate, however it makes no representation or warranty to this effect. You rely on this publication at your own risk. Royal Adelaide Hospital disclaims all liability for any claims, losses, damages, costs and expenses suffered or incurred as a result of reliance of this publication. As the information in this publication is subject to review, please contact a medical or health professional before using this publication.

half-life. However, half-lives vary between patients; various opioid doses may have been given during surgery; pain immediately after surgery may differ from pain later in the ward (e.g. shoulder-tip pain after laparoscopy or abdominal colic may have abated); sedation after anesthesia may have limited the amount of opioid given; and the volume status of the patient may have altered (hypovolemia reduces the amount of opioid needed). These and other variables make this calculation a guide at best.

Monitoring

Sedation scores, pain scores and respiratory rates should be monitored frequently, and hourly intervals are suggested.

Alterations of infusion rates

Because of the time taken for any alteration in infusion rate to have an effect, if analgesia is inadequate IV bolus doses should again be used to achieve patient comfort before the infusion rate is increased.

If an infusion is stopped it also takes five half-lives of the drug to return to a blood concentration of zero. Therefore if a patient becomes oversedated, the infusion should cease until they are more awake (sedation score <2), not merely be reduced to a lower rate.

Rectal route

The submucosal venous plexus of the rectum drains into the superior, middle and inferior rectal veins. Drug absorbed from the lower half of the rectum will pass into the latter two veins and into the inferior vena cava, thereby bypassing the portal vein and first-pass metabolism in the liver. This is one of the advantages of this route of administration. Drug absorbed through the rectal mucosa of the upper part of the rectum passes into the superior rectal vein and enters the portal system.

Rectal absorption is often variable owing to differences in the site of placement of the drug, the contents of the rectum and its blood supply. In addition, there is not always widespread patient – or staff – acceptance of this route of administration. Pat ient consent should be obtained before rectal administration of any drug, whether given awake or under anesthesia.

Rectal administration of drugs should be avoided in patients with pre-existing rectal lesions or who are immunosuppressed, and following some types of colorectal surgery.

In most instances similar doses of oral and rectal opioids are used, although there may be differences in bioavailability and rate of absorption for the reasons outlined above. The drug may not be distributed evenly throughout the suppository, and therefore doses of 'half a suppository' may not deliver half of the amount of opioid in that suppository.

Transdermal route

The stratum corneum of the epidermis forms a major barrier to the entry of drugs. However, opioids that are lipid soluble may be absorbed through the skin. Both fentanyl and buprenorphine are available as transdermal preparations.

Skin permeability can be affected by a number of factors, such as age, skin temperature, body site and ethnic group. Variations in these factors could lead to unpredictable rates of drug transfer across the skin. To minimize the influence of variable skin transfer, previously available (passive) transdermal delivery systems incorporated a membrane that is much less permeable than skin. This then became the rate-controlling step and ensured a more predictable rate of drug transfer.

Rate-controlling membrane patches have been widely used for many years, but have recently been replaced in most countries by transdermal therapeutic matrix systems. The opioid (fentanyl or buprenorphine) is dissolved in an adhesive matrix to form a drug-in-adhesive layer which, together with the stratum corneum, provides the rate-controlling function in the percutaneous absorption of the opioid. There is no drug reservoir or rate-controlling membrane.

The amount of drug delivered by the new patches is proportional to the surface area of the patch. They offer several advantages over the older reservoir systems, being smaller, thinner and more flexible, with better skin adherence over a 72-hour period, and are less likely to cause skin sensitization.

For fentanyl, the new patches show equivalence in bioavailability and pharmacokinetic profile to the earlier reservoir patches.

Transdermal fentanyl patches are available in sizes ranging from 2.1 mg up to 16.8 mg. These release the drug at a constant rate of about 12 μg/h to 100 μg/h, depending on patch size, for periods of 48–72 hours. These rates may vary markedly between patients. Once the patch is placed on the patient there is rapid absorption of the fentanyl into the skin reservoir because of the large concentration gradient between the two. The drug is then released more slowly from the skin, and it may be 17–48 hours before peak blood concentrations are reached. Similarly, if the patch is removed, the depot of fentanyl in the skin reservoir means that blood levels will decrease only slowly (the apparent elimination half-life is 13–25 hours).

Transdermal buprenorphine patches are also available in a variety of sizes, from 5 mg to 40 mg. They release the drug at constant rates of between 5 μg/h and 70 μg/h, depending on the size of the patch and the manufacturer.

Fentanyl patches are usually replaced every 72 hours. The low-dose buprenorphine patches (up to 20 μg/h) last for 7 days, whereas the higher-dose patches are usually changed every 3.5 days. It should be remembered that a significant amount of drug remains in the patch after removal, and caution must be taken with its disposal. For example, with the fentanyl transdermal system a 16.8 mg (16 800 μg) patch delivers 100 μg/h, which over 72 hours is 7200 μg, so the patch may still contain about 9600 μg (or the equivalent of around 500 mg morphine) after it is removed from the patient.

Transdermal fentanyl and buprenorphine patches are commonly used in the management of cancer and chronic pain. Fentanyl patches have not been found to be suitable for routine acute pain management: the slow onset of action does not allow for easy titration to analgesic effect and the incidence of respiratory depression is reported to be high. In addition, the continuation of effect even when the patch is removed means that any side effects that do occur may persist for some time. Severe complications, including death, have been reported with the inappropriate use of transdermal fentanyl in acute pain settings, and in many countries the use of fentanyl patches for the management of acute pain is specifically contraindicated. Transdermal buprenorphine patches are also not considered suitable.

A newer method of transdermal delivery, called *iontophoresis*, effects a more rapid transfer of drug through the skin by the application of an external electric field. It may also allow the rate of administration to be varied. It is not yet in common clinical use, although transdermal fentanyl PCA systems are now available in some countries (see Chapter 8).

Transmucosal routes

Transmucosal administration is the delivery of a drug through nasal, sublingual, buccal or pulmonary mucosal membranes. Recreational abusers of drugs have used the transmucosal route for many years, but it is not commonly utilized in clinical pain management. It is particularly suited to the more lipid-soluble opioids such as fentanyl, sufentanil, alfentanil and diamorphine. It has the advantage of avoiding first-pass metabolism (i.e. the drug enters the systemic circulation without first passing through the liver).

Intranasal

The human nasal mucosa contains drug-metabolizing enzymes, but whether the extent of nasal first-pass metabolism is of any clinical significance is unknown. It is has been suggested that the volume of a dose of any drug given intranasally should not exceed 150μL, in order to avoid excessive run-off into the pharynx.

Fentanyl, sufentanil, alfentanil, butorphanol, oxycodone, buprenorphine, diamorphine and pethidine (meperidine) are among the opioids that have been administered as a nasal spray. The method seems to be best suited to the more lipid-soluble opioids such fentanyl, sufentanil and alfentanil, when the resultant analgesia is said to be not just as effective but almost as fast in onset as similar doses of the drugs given by the IV route. In the case of fentanyl, peak blood concentrations may be reached in as little as 5 minutes.

Intranasal opioids can also be administered in metered doses, which can be 'patient controlled'. However, the systems used for delivery may allow ready and unauthorized access to the drugs.

Sublingual and buccal (oromucosal)

Fentanyl 'lollipops' (oral transmucosal fentanyl citrate, OTFC) that allow absorption from the oral mucosa are available in some countries and are used for anesthetic premedication and conscious sedation in monitored settings, primarily in children. They have also been used for 'breakthrough' analgesia in opioid-tolerant patients with cancer.

The use of OTFC in the management of acute and postoperative pain has not been adequately evaluated, and it is currently not recommended for pain relief in this setting. There is a risk of high peak plasma levels with unsupervised administration; in some countries it is specifically contraindicated for the treatment of acute pain.

Buprenorphine is used as an analgesic agent and also, increasingly, as an alternative to methadone in the treatment of heroin addiction. It is administered sublingually as a tablet and has a long duration of action (mean half-life 35 hours).

Pulmonary

Inhalational administration (as a nebulized aerosol) of some opioids, including morphine, diamorphine, fentanyl and hydromorphone, has been used in palliative care for the provision of analgesia and for the symptomatic control of breathlessness. Although with newer delivery systems the bioavailability of the drugs can be quite high, the unpredictable and large variation in absorption probably makes this route unsuitable for the management of acute pain.

Key points

Evidence level

II Intermittent subcutaneous morphine injections are as effective as intramuscular injections and have better patient acceptance

IV Continuous intravenous infusion of opioids in the general ward setting is associated with an increased risk of respiratory depression compared to other methods of parenteral opioid administration

IV Transdermal fentanyl should not be used in the management of acute pain because of safety concerns and difficulties in short-term dose adjustments needed for titration

Clinical practice points

Other than in the treatment of severe acute pain, and provided there are no contraindications to its use, the oral route is the route of choice for the administration of most analgesic drugs

Titration of opioids for severe acute pain is best achieved using intermittent intravenous bolus doses, as these allow more rapid titration of effect and avoid the uncertainty of drug absorption by other routes

Controlled-release opioid preparations should only be given at set intervals

The use of controlled-release opioid preparations as the sole agents for the early management of acute pain is discouraged because of difficulties in short-term dose adjustments needed for titration

Reproduced with permission from Acute Pain Management: Scientific Evidence ANZCA and FPM (2005)

References and further reading

Aronoff GM, Brennan MJ, Pritchard DD. (2005) Evidence-based oral transmucosal fentanyl citrate (OTFC) dosing guidelines. Pain Medicine 6: 305–14.

Australian and New Zealand College of Anaesthetists, Faculty of Pain Medicine (ANZCA, FPM). Acute Pain Management: Scientific Evidence, 2nd edn. Melbourne: Australian and New Zealand College of Anaesthetists, 2005. Also available online at: *http://www.anzca.edu.au/publications/acutepain.htm and http://www7.health.gov.au/nhmrc/publications/synopses/cp104syn.htm*

Breivik EK, Bjornsson GA, Skovlund E. (2000) A comparison of pain rating scales by sampling from clinical trial data. Clinical Journal of Pain 16: 22–8.

Cooper IM. (1996) Morphine for postoperative analgesia: a comparison of intramuscular and subcutaneous routes of administration. Anaesthesia and Intensive Care 24: 574–8.

Dale O, Hjortkjaer R, Kharasch ED. (2002) Nasal administration of opioids for pain management in adults. Acta Anaesthesiologica Scandinavica 46: 759–70.

Evans HC, Easthope SE. (2003) Transdermal buprenorphine. Drugs 63: 1999–2010.

Jeal W, Benfield P. (1997) Transdermal fentanyl: a review of its pharmacological properties and therapeutic efficacy in pain control. Drugs 53: 109–38.

Freynhagen R, von Giesen HJ, Busche P et al. (2005) Switching from reservoir to matrix systems for the transdermal delivery of fentanyl: a prospective, multi-center pilot study in outpatients with chronic pain. Journal of Pain and Symptom Management 30: 289–97.

Grond S, Radbruch L, Lehmann KA. (2000) Clinical pharmacokinetics of transdermal opioids: focus on transdermal fentanyl. Clinical Pharmacokinetics 38: 59–89.

Gould TH, Crosby DL, Harmer M et al. (1992) Policy for controlling pain after surgery: effect of sequential changes in management. British Medical Journal 305: 1187–93.

Lasagna L, Beecher HK. (1954) The optimal dose of morphine. Journal of the American Medical Association 156: 230–4.

Macintyre PE, Jarvis DA. (1996) Age is the best predictor of postoperative morphine requirements. Pain 64: 357–64.

Mildh LH, Leino KA, Kirvela OA. (1999) Effects of tramadol and meperidine on respiration, plasma catecholamine concentrations, and hemodynamics. Journal of Clinical Anesthesia 11: 310–16.

Peng WH, Sandler AN. (1999) A review of the use of fentanyl analgesia in the management of acute pain in adults. Anesthesiology 90: 576–99.

Schug SA, Torrie J. (1993) Safety assessment of postoperative pain management by an acute pain service. Pain 55: 387–91.

Semple TJ, Upton RN, Macintyre PE et al. (1997). Morphine blood concentrations in elderly postoperative patients following administration via an indwelling subcutaneous catheter. Anaesthesia 52: 318–23.

Sittl R, Griessinger N, Likar R. (2003) Analgesic efficacy and tolerability of transdermal buprenorphine in patients with inadequately controlled chronic pain related to cancer and other disorders: a multicenter, randomized, double-blind, placebo-controlled trial. Clinical Therapeutics 25: 150–68.

Patient-controlled analgesia

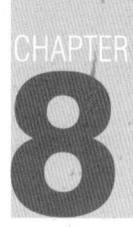

The words 'patient-controlled analgesia' (PCA) are commonly used to describe a method of pain relief that uses electronic or disposable infusion devices and allows patients to self-administer analgesic drugs (usually opioids) as required. However, in its broadest sense the phrase should not be restricted to a single route or method of analgesic administration, or to a single class of drug. It should refer to a general process that allows patients to determine when and how much analgesic medication they receive, regardless of the drug or route used.

This chapter deals primarily with intravenous (IV) PCA, although PCA via other systemic routes is also discussed. Patient-controlled epidural and other regional analgesia are covered in Chapters 9 and 10, respectively. The principles of PCA management are similar regardless of the route used.

Compared with conventional opioid analgesia (IM, SC or IV), IV PCA results in better pain relief and greater patient satisfaction, without increasing the incidence of opioid-related side effects.

The reasons for better analgesia may include:

- The intensity of acute pain is rarely constant and PCA means that small and frequent intravenous bolus doses of opioid can be given whenever the patient becomes uncomfortable, enabling individual titration of pain relief according to the degree of pain the patient is experiencing. Patients are more likely to be able to maintain blood concentrations of opioid within the therapeutic range ('analgesic corridor') (Figure 8.1).
- This flexibility helps to overcome the wide interpatient variation in opioid requirements (eight- to tenfold) in each age group (see Chapter 4).
- Patients are also able to titrate the amount of opioid delivered against dose-related side effects.

Equipment

There are two basic types of PCA device. Each has two components, a reservoir and a patient-control module.

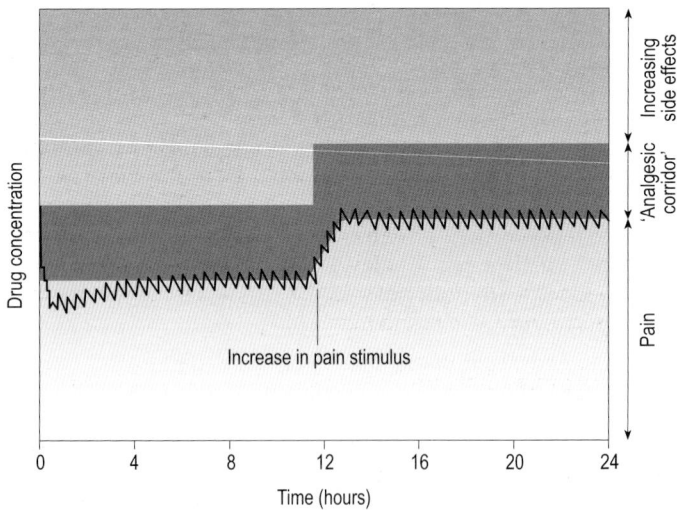

Figure 8.1 Patient-controlled analgesia is more likely to keep blood concentrations of opioid within the 'analgesic corridor' and allows rapid titration if there is an increase in pain stimulus that requires higher blood levels of opioid in order to maintain analgesia.

Electronic syringe pumps

Electronic PCA machines have been commercially available since the early 1970s. Within preset limits, they deliver a bolus dose of drug when the patient presses a demand button connected to the pump. Access to the syringe (or other drug reservoir) and the microprocessor program are only possible using a key or access code. Certain variables are prescribed and programmed into the machine (see below) and control how much drug the patient can receive. Most machines can also deliver a continuous or background infusion, thus PCA machines can operate in three modes:

- PCA mode only
- Continuous infusion only
- A combination of PCA with a continuous (background) infusion.

Patients using PCA mode are instructed to push the demand button whenever they are uncomfortable. If the machine has a pneumatic demand mechanism and the patient is unable to use either hand, a length of plastic tubing can be attached to the machine instead of the hand-held button and the patient is instructed to blow into this tubing. Some machines will also operate with a pressure-sensitive pad or foot pedal. These alternative aids may be particularly useful for patients with conditions such as quadriplegia, widespread burns involving the hands and arms, or severe rheumatoid arthritis.

The inherent safety of the technique lies in the fact that, as long as the machine is in PCA mode only (i.e. there is no continuous infusion), further doses of opioid will not be delivered should the patient become excessively sedated, because no further demands will be made. This assumes that the patient is the only one pressing the button. In a general ward setting especially, staff should explain to the patient, relatives and friends that no one but the patient is allowed to operate the PCA machine.

In some settings (e.g. pediatric or intensive care) use by someone other than the patient may be allowed in some circumstances. However, such use will reduce the inherent safety of PCA and must be accompanied by appropriate instructions and monitoring.

Disposable PCA devices

A number of disposable PCA devices have been developed. Many deliver a fixed volume of drug following each demand. In some devices, increases or decreases in the size of the incremental bolus dose can be accomplished by changing the concentration of drug in the reservoir. In others, such as the transdermal system described later, the dose cannot be changed. Another potential problem with disposable devices is that the drug reservoir is more easily accessible than in locked electronic devices, and the security of controlled drugs may therefore be compromised. In addition, unlike with electronic pumps, there is no administration history.

Consumables

One-way antireflux and antisiphon valves are recommended for use with PCA and are suggested whenever a syringe pump is used to deliver other drugs, such as ketamine or epidural local anesthetic/opioid solutions. Antireflux valves prevent opioid backing up into the primary IV line should the IV cannula become occluded, so that delivery of multiple doses does not occur if the occlusion is cleared. They should therefore be mandatory unless the PCA is connected to the patient via a dedicated IV line. Antisiphon valves, placed between the syringe (or other drug reservoir) and the patient, will prevent siphoning (emptying by gravity) of the drug reservoir if it is above the level of the patient and not properly fixed in the machine, or if the reservoir develops an air leak (e.g. due to a cracked syringe).

Analgesic and other drugs used with PCA

Opioids

Many opioids have been used with PCA (morphine being the most common), but those having very short (e.g. alfentanil, remifentanil) or very long (e.g. methadone) durations of action are not usually recommended, at least for general ward use. Partial agonist or agonist–antagonist opioids are used far less commonly than pure opioid agonists.

There is little evidence to suggest major differences in either efficacy or side effects between the opioids commonly used for PCA, although patients may report more pruritus with morphine. However, if drug-related side effects fail to respond to specific treatment, some patients may benefit if a change to another opioid is made (opioid rotation).

In patients with renal impairment the use of a drug with no active metabolites, such as fentanyl, might be preferred. Norpethidine (normeperidine) toxicity can occur even in the absence of renal problems and within 24 hours of starting therapy. As the aim of PCA is to allow patients to determine the amount of opioid they need, and as the doses required to achieve adequate analgesia are unpredictable and vary enormously between patients, it is probably best to avoid the use of pethidine (meperidine) with PCA.

Other drugs

This chapter focuses on the use of opioids with PCA. Much less often, combinations of an opioid with another drug are used. Examples include the addition of ketamine or clonidine, in attempts to improve pain relief, or of droperidol for the prevention or treatment of nausea and vomiting. However, large interpatient variations in PCA opioid requirements mean that patients are likely to receive very widely varying doses of the added drug. This could lead to an inadequate effect of the added drug in some patients and an excessive effect in others.

The PCA 'prescription'

There are many different models of microprocessor-controlled PCA machine now available. Although the variables that can be programmed into the machines might differ a little between devices, a number of features are common to most. Commonly used settings for IV PCA variables are listed in Box 8.1.

Loading dose

Patient-controlled analgesia is a maintenance therapy. That is, it is a good way to maintain patient comfort but an ineffective way of achieving that comfort in the first place. It may not be effective if moderate or severe pain is present at commencement. To make the patient comfortable before PCA is started, a loading dose of opioid is needed. There is an enormous interpatient variation in the amount of opioid required as a loading dose and it is usually better to individualize this dose for each patient prior to starting PCA (e.g. by using the protocols in Chapter 7) rather than program a single loading dose via the PCA machine.

After regional anesthesia moderate to severe pain can occur rapidly as the local anesthetic block wears off. The use of PCA alone may be ineffective in controlling this pain, and a method to load the patient must be available even if the patient has returned to the ward after surgery.

Incremental (bolus) dose

The bolus dose is the amount of opioid (in milligrams or micrograms) that the PCA machine will deliver when the demand button is pressed. The size of the incremental dose, along with the lockout interval (see below), can influence the success or otherwise of PCA. If the dose is too small, patients will not be able to obtain adequate analgesia and may then question the efficacy of the drug or technique. If the dose is too large, the administration of a single dose will result in adverse effects, which may then discourage ongoing use of PCA.

Box 8.1

Commonly prescribed initial variables for IV PCA in opioid-naive patients

Variable	Value		Comments
Loading dose	0 mg (ie. zero)		Patients should be comfortable before PCA is started, and therefore it is best to titrate opioid analgesia for each patient before starting PCA
Bolus dose	Morphine	1 mg	In patients aged 70 or older, consider reducing doses by 50%
	Fentanyl	20 µg	
	Hydromorphone	200 µg	Bolus dose may need to be increased if analgesia is inadequate
	Tramadol	10–20 mg	
Concentration	Morphine	1 mg/mL	Best if standardized for each drug
	Fentanyl	20 µg/mL	
	Hydromorphone	200 µg/mL	
	Tramadol	10 mg/mL	
Dose duration	Cannot be adjusted in most PCA machines, but where this can be done, 'stat' (delivers 1 mL over approximately 30 s) is the shortest dose duration		
Lockout	5–8 min		Not worth altering (no evidence to show any benefit)
Background infusion	0 mg/h (i.e. zero)		Not used routinely in opioid-naive patients (see text) If prescribed, it may be appropriate to use a rate of infusion in mg/h that is no greater than the size of the bolus dose in mg
1-h or 4-h limits			Consider omitting (no evidence to show any benefit)

Commonly used initial dose sizes (in opioid-naive patients) are given in Box 8.1. The optimal incremental dose for each patient is one that results in good pain relief with minimal side effects. Therefore, adjustments to the size of the initial dose may be required, so that PCA can be better tailored to the individual patient.

With conventional intermittent opioid regimens the dose prescribed should be reduced as the age of the patient increases. As patients using PCA can vary the total daily dose according to the number of demands made, a progressive decrease in dose with increasing age is not necessary. However, patients over 70 have, on average, less than half the total daily opioid requirement of a 20-year-old. Therefore it is reasonable to start with smaller incremental doses (see Chapter 14). Patients who are opioid-tolerant (see Chapter 14) may require significantly higher bolus doses than these to achieve adequate analgesia.

Dose duration

The rate at which the PCA machine delivers the bolus dose can be altered in some machines, allowing the dose to be delivered as a short infusion (e.g. over 5 minutes). If subcutaneous PCA is used (see later), rapid delivery of a dose may cause some stinging; a slower rate of delivery will reduce the chance of this occurring.

Lockout interval

The time from the *end* of the delivery of one dose until the machine will respond to another demand is called the lockout interval. This plays a key part in increasing the safety of PCA, as it allows the patient to feel the effect of one dose before receiving a subsequent one. Practically, however, lockout intervals of 5–8 minutes are commonly prescribed, regardless of the opioid used, even though it may take up to 15 minutes or longer for the peak effect of an IV dose of morphine (most commonly used in PCA) to be seen. A longer lockout interval reduces the ability of the patient to rapidly titrate the amount of opioid required and may decrease the effectiveness of PCA.

When patients are told about the lockout interval, it is important to ensure that they realize it only means that another dose *can* be delivered, should they press the button, and not that they *need* to press every 5–8 minutes.

Lockout intervals of 5–8 minutes mean that, allowing for time for the dose to be delivered, a patient could demand and receive up to ten doses of opioid each hour. In reality, if patients feel that a particular incremental dose is not effective, they will not continue to press the demand button. Most patients have an inherent maximum frequency of demand, and it is uncommon for someone to sustain a demand rate of more than three or four doses per hour. If analgesia is inadequate, despite an average of three or four doses each hour, it may be preferable to increase the size of the bolus dose rather than reduce the lockout interval or instruct the patient to press the button more often.

Continuous (background) infusion

Most PCA machines can deliver a continuous infusion. Used at a low rate in addition to PCA mode (patient demand mode), it was hoped that a continuous infusion would lead to a constant but subanalgesic blood concentration, and that this would enable the patient to make fewer demands, sleep for longer periods and wake in less pain.

Unfortunately, the routine addition of a continuous infusion does not have the beneficial effects that were anticipated for the average patient. Instead, it:

- does not always reduce the number of demands made by the patient;
- may increase the total amount of opioid delivered;
- does not always result in better analgesia;
- does not always result in improved sleep patterns;
- significantly increases the risk of respiratory depression.

A continuous infusion reduces the inherent safety of the PCA technique, as opioid will be delivered regardless of the sedation level of the patient.

Although the routine use of a background infusion is not recommended, it may be required in some opioid-naive patients (see below) and, more commonly, in those who are opioid tolerant (see Chapter 14).

Example

An opioid-naive patient has used 100 mg morphine in the previous 24 hours and is complaining of repeatedly waking in severe pain. An increase in the size of the bolus dose to 2 mg has not helped.

100 mg in 24 hours   = 4 mg/h (approx)

50% of 4 mg/h   = 2 mg/h

∴ Background infusion = 2 mg/h

Opioid-naive patients

There may be some benefit from the use of a continuous infusion in patients who have high opioid requirements or who complain of waking repeatedly in severe pain at night. In both these situations the daytime opioid requirement of the patient is known and the rate of infusion can be adjusted accordingly. A typical approach is to order a continuous infusion that provides about 50% of a patient's *known* hourly opioid dose. If the combination of a continuous infusion and PCA mode is prescribed in opioid-naive patients, it is recommended that the rate in milligrams per hour should usually not exceed the size of the bolus dose in milligrams.

In acute pain management daily opioid requirements often decrease rapidly, therefore the need for the infusion, as well as the rate of infusion prescribed, should be reassessed frequently.

Opioid-tolerant patients

In patients who are opioid-tolerant background infusions may sometimes be used in place of their normal (preadmission) opioid requirements (see Chapter 14).

Concentration

For consistency and safety, each institution should standardize the concentrations of drugs administered by PCA where possible. Some manufacturers of PCA machines suggest that the volume delivered following each demand should not be less than 0.5 mL. The smaller the volume of the bolus dose, the greater number of doses required to trigger the occlusion alarm should IV access become obstructed.

Dose limits

Hourly or 4-hourly dose limits prevent the patient receiving more than a designated amount of opioid within a set time. However, large inter-patient variations in opioid requirements make it impossible to predict the 'safe' limit for each patient. For example, a commonly prescribed limit is 30 mg of morphine (or equianalgesic doses of an alternative opioid) in 4 hours. This may be inadequate for some patients, yet may be all that an older patient requires in 24 hours.

For PCA to be used effectively, a wide range of opioid doses will be required. The setting of a dose limit may not mean added safety for patients with low opioid requirements and may prevent those needing higher doses from obtaining good pain relief. The amount of opioid a patient is 'allowed' should not be influenced by preconceived ideas of maximum doses. In general, patients have not received an excessive dose if they remain unsedated.

There is no evidence of any benefit that can be attributed to these dose limits. The setting of a limit could give staff a false sense of security, as they may believe that the patient cannot receive an excessive dose of drug. As with other features designed to increase patient safety with PCA, the setting of a dose limit cannot compensate for any shortcomings in monitoring. Hourly or 4-hourly limits are not present on all machines.

Requirements for the safe management of PCA

Suitable patient

The 'suitable' patient is one who is happy to take some control of their pain relief, wants to use PCA, and can understand how it is to be used. The majority of patients appreciate the control that PCA gives them, the ability to rapidly titrate their own analgesia and to balance acceptable pain relief with the severity of any side effects that may occur, and not having to wait for analgesic medications or bother nursing staff. These are probably some of the reasons that patients using PCA sometimes express a greater satisfaction with this technique than with others such as epidural analgesia, even though the degree of pain relief may be less. Some patients may not want this control and would prefer the nursing and medical staff to manage their pain relief.

Safety and efficacy require the patient to have an adequate understanding of the PCA technique. Although very young and very old patients may be less likely to manage PCA successfully, it should not be withheld simply on these grounds. Many children as young as 4 years old, as well as patients in their 90s, may cope with PCA very well as long as they understand the explanations given and are willing to be active participants in their own care. Similarly, patients should not automatically be excluded from consideration if there is mild mental impairment or a language barrier. Relatives or translators can be asked to interpret verbal instructions, and patient education leaflets can be written in many languages. If staff feel that despite these measures the patient still does not understand PCA, alternative methods of pain relief will be needed. Patients who have preoperative evidence of dementia are often not suitable for PCA, and those who become confused may need to have PCA discontinued.

Some patients and/or their relatives and friends may be concerned about the risk of overdose or addiction, or do not trust the PCA machine. Appropriate education, both before and during PCA use, will usually help overcome these fears.

Addiction to opioids was once considered to be a contraindication for the use of PCA. However, as these patients may have very high and unpredictable opioid requirements, PCA is a very useful method of pain relief (see Chapter 14).

Trained nursing and medical staff

PCA is an effective way of providing good pain relief, but the results depend on a good understanding of the technique. Therefore, PCA should only be used by medical and nursing staff who have the appropriate training. An inadequate understanding of PCA, the drugs and doses used, the monitoring requirements and the management of common problems can, at worst, increase the risk of complications. At best, it can prove to be a very expensive way of providing suboptimal analgesia.

Nursing education and accreditation programs that have to be completed by each nurse before he or she can take responsibility for a patient with PCA are recommended. If this is done, nursing staff may be able to program PCA machines, change syringes and make alterations to the program according to the PCA standard orders.

In many institutions the use of PCA is supervised by an acute pain service.

Standard orders

To maximize the effectiveness of PCA and minimize the risk of complications, standard orders and nursing procedure protocols are recommended. However, even when these are used, PCA may be more effective when supervised by an acute pain service team than by less experienced medical staff.

To standardize orders throughout the institution, preprinted forms are suggested. Examples of preprinted PCA standard order forms are given at the end of this chapter.

Standard orders can be a safe and effective way of initiating treatment with PCA. However, the orders may not be suitable for all patients. Regular evaluation will allow appropriate alterations to be made so that maximum therapeutic benefit can be obtained with minimum possible side effects. Assessment should usually include:

- Effectiveness of analgesia at rest and with activity;
- Effectiveness of the treatment of any side effects;
- An overall assessment of the patient, including the possibility of non-PCA-related complications and any concurrent medication orders.

Standard orders need to cover the following areas.

Non-drug treatment orders

Non-drug treatment orders may include a statement to eliminate the concurrent ordering of CNS depressants or other opioids by unauthorized medical staff; orders for oxygen; the need for one-way antireflux and antisiphon valves; and instructions on whom to contact should problems occur.

Monitoring and documentation requirements

As with any opioid regimen used for the management of acute pain, the pain score, sedation score and respiratory rate should be monitored. These should be recorded at regular intervals, along with the total amount of opioid delivered, the dose of any drug administered for the treatment of side effects, and any changes that have been made to the PCA program.

The monitoring and recording of these parameters allows a regular assessment of the progress of each patient and for rational changes to be made to PCA orders so that treatment is individualized. It should be noted that most patients will titrate their pain relief to a level at which they are comfortable and not aim for complete analgesia, even in the absence of opioid-related side effects.

Certain higher-risk patients, such as the morbidly obese and those with sleep apnea or severe pulmonary disease, may require additional and closer observation.

PCA orders

All variables of the PCA program need to be prescribed (see Box 8.1). Also, it might be helpful, in some settings, to have orders that enable staff to increase or reduce the size of the bolus dose (within set limits) if needed.

Orders for the treatment of side effects

The inclusion of standardized orders for the recognition and management of opioid-related side effects will minimize delays in treatment.

Nursing procedure protocols

The format of nursing procedure protocols for PCA will vary with each institution, but key elements include:

- The institution's policy on accreditation (credentialing) of nursing staff;
- The mechanisms for checking and discarding PCA opioids;
- Monitoring and documentation requirements;
- Instructions for:
  - checking the PCA settings against the prescription (e.g. at the change of each shift);
  - checking the amount of drug delivered (from the infusion pump display) against the amount remaining in the drug reservoir;
  - the setting up and programming of PCA pumps;
  - the use of antireflux and antisiphon valves,
  - management of equipment faults and alarms.

Management of inadequate analgesia

Inadequate analgesia may occur for a number of reasons, including an inadequate loading dose, inappropriate patient use, the presence of opioid-related side effects and ineffective PCA prescriptions. Suggestions for the management of inadequate analgesia are summarized in Box 8.2.

Inadequate loading dose

Patients must be given an adequate loading dose before PCA is started. This is essential, as trying to establish analgesia or to rectify inadequate analgesia is difficult or often impossible with PCA alone. In addition, if a patient is noted to have inadequate analgesia at any time during PCA treatment, 'reloading' may be needed.

Inadequate bolus dose

Standard orders are designed for the 'average' patient, and in some cases the usual incremental bolus dose may be suboptimal. If PCA does not seem to be providing satisfactory analgesia it is worth looking at the number of doses the patient has received over the previous few hours. If this is fewer than two per hour on average, further instruction is probably needed and the patient should be encouraged to use PCA more often. On the other hand, a patient who is already receiving three or more doses each hour cannot always be expected to maintain or increase that demand rate, and it may be reasonable to increase the size of the bolus dose by 50–100%.

Before the bolus dose is increased, the patient should be reviewed. Increasing pain, increasing analgesic requirements, or pain out of

---

Box 8.2

Management of inadequate analgesia*

- Reassess the patient
  - consider another cause for new or increased pain, such as the development of a postoperative or post-injury complication that might require treatment
  - if the pain is poorly responsive to opioids (e.g. neuropathic pain) other treatment options may be required
  - treat opioid-related side effects as needed
- Check that other components of multimodal analgesia (i.e. paracetamol or NSAIDs) have been given
- Give additional opioid to 'reload' the patient if needed
- If the patient is receiving two bolus doses/h or fewer (average), re-educate the patient and encourage more frequent use of the demand button
- If the patient is receiving three or more doses/h (average), the size of the bolus dose may need to be increased
- If the patient cannot use the hand-held demand button, alternative mechanisms can be used):
  - foot pedal-activated
  - breath-activated (Note: a filter should be placed in-line between the patient and the PCA machine)

* These strategies are suggestions only and may not be needed in, or be suitable for, the treatment of all patients.

---

proportion to the procedure or number of days elapsed since injury or postoperatively, requires a reassessment of the patient. There may be another cause for the pain, for example the development of a complication (e.g. a compartment syndrome following limb injury, or a leaking anastomosis following bowel surgery). The pain may not be completely responsive to opioids: colicky abdominal pain may respond better to an anticholinergic agent or peppermint water, and pain following nerve injury to a drug such as amitriptyline.

'Successful' and 'unsuccessful' demands

Many PCA machines are able to record the numbers of both 'successful' (when a dose was delivered) and 'unsuccessful' (when the button was pressed during the lockout interval) demands. Unfortunately, this does not always reflect the true analgesic requirement of the patient. Some patients, like some people waiting at elevators or traffic lights, will always press the button a number of times in rapid succession although they only want the result of a single press.

Patients with higher ratings for anxiety and depression have also been shown to make more demands but do not always require more opioid. High demand rates may also result from inappropriate patient or non-patient use (see above), as well as the onset of confusion; other explanations may be the use of a bolus dose that is too small, or poor opioid responsiveness of the pain.

Side effects

Patients who are experiencing nausea or vomiting, or other side effects they perceive to be due to the opioid, may be reluctant to continue with PCA. Staff should ensure that appropriate therapy for the side effects is given (see below). If these persist, a change to another opioid (an opioid rotation) may be effective.

'Step-down' analgesia

The importance of appropriate 'step-down' analgesia (that is, analgesia a patient is prescribed after PCA has been stopped) needs to be acknowledged. There is little point in trying to maximize patient comfort with PCA and then leaving them in significant discomfort when PCA is stopped, simply because adequate attention has not been paid to the subsequent pain relief regimen.

Opioid requirements during PCA can be used as guide to the appropriate 'step-down' regimen. If the patient is tolerating oral fluids, oral opioids can be ordered. If PCA is ceased before oral fluids can be given, other parenteral (IM, SC or IV) opioids will be needed. In general, PCA is usually continued at least until oral opioids can be used.

There should be some overlap of pain therapies so that the subsequent regimen has time to have an effect before PCA is stopped. If there is to be a change in clinician responsibility for the patient's pain management then this needs to be clearly understood by all staff.

Oral opioids

Any of the oral opioids suitable for the management of acute pain may be used following PCA (see Chapter 4). The oral dosage can be based on the amount of IV opioid used in the 24 hours prior to stopping PCA, and the equianalgesic doses of PCA and oral opioids.

Background analgesic agents such as non-steroidal anti-inflammatory drugs (NSAIDs) and paracetamol (acetaminophen), which should be part of the multimodal analgesic regimen including PCA, should be continued with the oral opioids. This will continue to reduce the amount of opioid required and they can be continued once opioids are no longer needed.

As the intensity of acute pain usually decreases daily, it is likely that the patient will require less opioid than would be expected based solely on equianalgesic doses. The oral regimen therefore needs to accommodate this expected decrease in dose requirement. For example, if oral oxycodone or tramadol is prescribed to follow IV morphine PCA, the daily requirements are likely to be less (based on the equianalgesic doses of 10 mg IV morphine = 20 mg oral oxycodone = 100 mg oral tramadol) than the previous 24-hour PCA morphine requirement. To enable patients to titrate their own analgesia, it may be appropriate to allow a daily oral dose range between 0.5 and 2 times the last 24-hour PCA morphine requirement.

Example

A patient has used 60 mg PCA morphine in the immediate last 24 hours.

60 mg morphine in 24 hrs = 60 mg oxycodone in next 24 hours (approx)

∴ daily oxycodone range = 30–120 mg (5–20 mg every 4 hours)

∴ oxycodone order = '5–20 mg 1–2 hourly PRN'

OR tramadol order = '50–100 mg 1–2 hourly PRN'

Depending on clinical circumstances, the oral opioid may be ordered on a PRN or time-contingent basis. The 'PCA principle' should continue and patients should, in most cases, have some input into the dose given and the timing of that dose.

Some suggested oxycodone dose ranges based on prior PCA use are outlined in Box 8.3.

Intramuscular or subcutaneous opioids

To convert PCA requirements to an intermittent intramuscular (IM) or subcutaneous (SC) regimen the 24-hour PCA dose can be divided by 8 to find an appropriate dose range. Although division by 8 estimates a 3-hourly dose, it is reasonable to add additional flexibility by ordering the range of doses 2-hourly PRN (see Chapter 4).

Example

A patient has used 60 mg PCA morphine in the immediate last 24 hours.

60 mg PCA morphine in 24 hours = 60 mg SC morphine in next 24 hours (approx) = 7.5 mg 3-hourly

∴ SC morphine order = '5–10 mg 2-hourly PRN'

Box 8.3

Examples of calculations for immediate-release oral oxycodone to follow IV PCA morphine

Immediate last 24-h IV PCA morphine dose	Oral oxycodone ordered '2-hourly PRN'
30 mg	5–10 mg
45 mg	5–15 mg
60 mg	5–20 mg
75 mg	5–25 mg
90 mg	10–30 mg

* These doses are suggestions only and may not be needed in, or be suitable for, the treatment of all patients.

Complications of PCA

Complications of PCA may be related to the side effects of the drugs used, the equipment involved, or management by staff or patients.

Side effects related to the opioid

Opioid-related side effects may develop regardless of the route of administration (see Chapter 2). Suggested options for the management of these side effects are summarized in Box 8.4.

Nausea and vomiting

If nausea or vomiting occurs an appropriate antiemetic should be given or, if that antiemetic appears to be ineffective, an alternative ordered. If a patient has low opioid requirements a decrease in the size of the bolus dose can also be tried. Patients who complain of a wave of nausea or dizziness a few minutes after pressing the demand button may benefit from a smaller bolus dose or a slower rate of infusion (i.e. an increase in the 'dose duration').

Although there is little evidence to support a difference in the incidence of nausea and vomiting with different opioids, individual patients may appear to be more sensitive to one particular drug. In this case, and if other measures have failed, a change to another opioid is worth considering. It may also be that the opioid is not the cause, or not the sole cause, of the nausea and vomiting (see Chapter 4).

Box 8.4

Management of side effects of PCA opioids*

Nausea/vomiting	Administer antiemetics and *add* additional antiemetics if ineffective
	If nausea seems related to the PCA demand, try reducing the size of the bolus dose (if requirements are low) or increasing the dose duration to 5 minutes
	Consider other possible causes (e.g. ileus)
	Change to another opioid
Pruritus	Check that pruritus is likely to be opioid related
	Consider a change to another opioid
	Although naloxone may relieve the pruritus, it may also reverse analgesia, especially if given in repeated doses.
	Antihistamines may not be effective, as the pruritus is thought to result from an action on opioid receptors rather than histamine release (see Chapter 4) and may increase the risk of sedation
Sedation/respiratory depression	Check no other reason for sedation (e.g. administration of a sedative)
	Sedation score = 2: respiratory rate ≥ 8/min: halve the bolus dose
	Sedation score = 2: respiratory rate < 8/min: halve the bolus dose. If close supervision of the patient is not possible, consider administration of naloxone 100 µg IV and repeat PRN
	Sedation score = 3 (regardless of respiratory rate): give naloxone 100 µg IV and repeat PRN; cease PCA until patient is more awake. Restart at half the dose
Urinary retention	Catheterize
Confusion	Probably not related to the PCA opioid; look for other possible causes (e.g. hypoxia, sepsis, alcohol or benzodiazepine withdrawal)
	PCA may need to be stopped and alternative analgesia organized

(Continued)

Box 8.4—cont'd

Management of side effects of PCA opioids*

Decreased bowel motility/colicky pain	Anticipatory treatment where possible Discourage use of PCA to cover discomfort resulting from resumption of peristalsis; if pain becomes severe, consider bowel obstruction. If treatment is needed, peppermint could be tried
Hypotension	Look for hypovolemia and other causes of hypotension

* These strategies are suggestions only and may not be needed in, or be suitable for, the treatment of all patients.

As the emetic effects of opioids are enhanced by vestibular stimulation, the patient may feel better lying flat and minimizing movement until any treatment has had time to have an effect.

Pruritus

As outlined in Chapter 4, pruritus may be due to histamine release or a consequence of possible μ opioid receptor activation. It is more common following morphine than pethidine (meperidine) or fentanyl.

After checking that any pruritus is likely to be due to the opioid (i.e. its distribution is over the face and trunk) and whether the patient is disturbed by this side effect, the safest treatment in the first instance is to change to another opioid, preferably fentanyl. Antihistamines, because of their sedative effects, may add to the risk of sedation and respiratory depression. Pruritus may also respond to small, carefully titrated doses of intravenous naloxone, but there is a risk that this may reverse the analgesia. Nalbuphine in small IV doses is also sometimes effective.

Sedation and respiratory depression

The best clinical indicator of early respiratory depression is sedation. If a patient has a sedation score of 2 (see Chapter 3) a reduction in the size of the PCA bolus dose (e.g. by 50%) is usually indicated. Even if sedatives have been given this may still be the safest course of action – the dose can always be increased again if analgesia is inadequate, once the patient is more alert.

If the patient has a sedation score of 2 and a respiratory rate below 8 per minute, the size of the bolus dose should also be reduced. Whether or not a small dose of naloxone (100 μg IV) is considered necessary in this instance may depend on factors such as staffing levels. If no nurse is available to keep a continued close watch on the patient, it may be safer to administer naloxone.

If a patient develops severe respiratory depression with a sedation score of 3 (difficult to rouse, or unrousable), naloxone should be given. Remember that naloxone has a shorter half-life than commonly used opioid agonists, and repeated doses or an infusion may be needed.

Respiratory depression during PCA therapy has been reported in patients following postoperative hemorrhage. A normally appropriate incremental dose of opioid may become excessive in the presence of hypovolemia. Until the patient is normovolemic, smaller incremental bolus doses may be needed.

Urinary retention

Urinary retention may occur as a result of opioid administration. Whatever the cause, the patient may need to be catheterized – either an 'in/out' or an indwelling catheter.

Confusion

Opioids will not usually be the cause, or the sole cause, of confusion. Other possible causes include hypoxemia, sepsis, other drugs (particularly those with anticholinergic side effects) and alcohol or drug withdrawal (see Chapter 14). Nevertheless, PCA may need to be discontinued as the patient may press the demand button inappropriately. Alternative methods of pain relief should then be organized.

Inhibition of bowel motility

To a greater or lesser extent inhibition of bowel motility is an inevitable consequence of the use of opioids. Where possible, and if opioids are to be used for some days, treatment should be anticipatory. Occasionally, patients may use PCA opioids to cover the often-vague abdominal discomfort ('windy pains' or 'gas cramps') related to the resumption of peristalsis, e.g. after abdominal surgery, but the use of opioids in this way will further inhibit the return of bowel function. The patient should be encouraged to mobilize rather than use PCA for this discomfort. If treatment is needed, peppermint may be as effective as anticholinergic drugs such as hyoscine, and have fewer side effects.

Hypotension

Opioids themselves do not usually cause hypotension, but may unmask an existing hypovolemia.

Masking of postoperative or post-injury complications

Concerns have been expressed about the risk of PCA 'masking' signs of a postoperative or post-injury complication (e.g. urinary retention, compartment syndrome, myocardial infarction and pulmonary embolus) and that patients will simply increase their PCA use to treat any 'new' pain without informing nursing or medical staff, resulting in a delay in diagnosis.

If the patient is monitored carefully, the risk of this occurring should be very low. Any unexpected increase in analgesic use, or the site, severity or character of the pain being treated, warrants careful assessment and investigation, as it may signal the development of a new surgical or medical diagnosis. Any adjustment to the PCA program should be made bearing the potential underlying problem in mind.

Complications related to equipment, staff or patients

Equipment malfunction

In the earlier years of PCA there were case reports of interference from current surges or static electricity leading to machine malfunction. Should this happen it will usually 'fail safe' – for example, the program will default to the lowest setting possible for a bolus dose. However, cases were recorded where malfunction led to the continuous delivery of the contents of a syringe. Although this problem appears to have been overcome in later machines, it may be wise to check the PCA program whenever the syringe is changed and whenever a machine is connected to or disconnected from mains power. Frayed wires in a patient-demand cable (connecting the demand button to the PCA machine) have led to short-circuiting and automatic, unintentional drug delivery.

Other equipment problems have included cracked syringe barrels, which have allowed the contents of the syringe to empty by gravity, and faulty one-way valves.

Staff error

Operator error can lead to misprogramming of the PCA machine, improper loading of the syringe or cassette, loading of the 'wrong' syringe (e.g. wrong drug or wrong concentration), and incorrect use of (or failure to use) antireflux or antisiphon one-way valves. Errors in PCA prescriptions have also occurred, either inadvertently or due to an inadequate knowledge of PCA. In addition, the inappropriate administration of sedative drugs or supplementary opioids by other routes has led to respiratory depression.

Inappropriate patient or non-patient use

Respiratory depression may occur if the patient does not adequately comprehend the PCA technique. Examples include pushing the demand button every time the lockout interval ends, or mistaking the button for a nurse-call button. It has also been reported following activation of PCA by well-meaning (or rarely not so well-meaning) relatives or friends, and hospital staff. If a patient using PCA is sedated but there is evidence of ongoing PCA demands, non-patient use should be excluded.

Tampering

Despite most PCA machines having a locked cover, the occasional patient has managed to extract the syringe without damaging the equipment.

Alternative systemic routes of PCA administration

Subcutaneous

A number of opioids have been administered by SC PCA, including morphine, fentanyl, diamorphine and hydromorphone. The resulting analgesia appears to be as effective as IV PCA, although the onset of analgesia will be slower. Use of SC PCA may be indicated if another drug that is incompatible with the opioid is running in the primary IV line, or if there is no IV access (even temporarily). Two suggestions for the management of subcutaneous PCA are outlined below.

1. The same drug and same concentration as for IV PCA can be used, but the following changes to the PCA program are suggested:
   - Double the bolus dose;
   - Double the lockout period to 10 minutes;
   - Where possible, increase the dose duration to 5 minutes.

2. The same drug in a stronger concentration can be used:
   - Increase the concentration by a factor of 5 (to reduce the volume infused into the subcutaneous tissue);
   - Double the bolus dose;
   - Double the lockout period to 10 minutes;
   - No change needs to be made to the dose duration.

Transmucosal and transdermal

Devices have also been developed or adapted to allow oral and intranasal opioid PCA. Iontophoretic transdermal fentanyl PCA patches are also now available in some countries. All may be as effective as IV PCA.

As yet, most are not widely used. Usually disposable, these devices will have the same potential disadvantages as other disposable PCA equipment: limited ability to alter the size of the bolus dose administered, and security issues relating to ease of access to the opioid reservoir.

Epidural and other regional analgesia

The epidural route can also be used for PCA. For further details see Chapters 9 and 10.

Key points

Evidence level

I Intravenous opioid PCA provides better analgesia than conventional parenteral opioid regimens

I Patient preference for intravenous PCA is higher than for conventional regimens

II There is little evidence that one opioid via PCA is superior to another with regards to analgesic or adverse effects in general; on an individual patient basis one opioid may be better tolerated than another

II The addition of a background infusion to IV PCA does not improve pain relief or sleep, or reduce the number of PCA demands

II Subcutaneous and intranasal PCA opioids can be as effective as IV PCA

IV The risk of respiratory depression with PCA is increased when a background infusion is used

Clinical practice points

Adequate analgesia needs to be obtained prior to commencement of PCA. Initial orders for bolus doses should take into account individual patient factors such as a history of prior opioid use and patient age. Individual PCA prescriptions may need to be adjusted

PCA infusion systems must incorporate antisiphon valves and in non-dedicated lines, antireflux valves.

Reproduced with permission from Acute Pain Management: Scientific Evidence ANZCA and FPM (2005)

References and further reading

Australian and New Zealand College of Anaesthetists, Faculty of Pain Medicine (ANZCA, FPM). Acute Pain Management: Scientific Evidence, 2nd edn. Melbourne: Australian and New Zealand College of Anaesthetists, 2005. Also available online at: *http://www.anzca.edu.au/publications/acutepain.htm* and *http://www7.health.gov.au/nhmrc/publications/synopses/cp104syn.htm*

Brandner B, Bromley L, Blagrove M. (2002) Influence of psychological factors in the use of patient controlled analgesia. Acute Pain 4: 53–6.

Cashman JN, Dolin SJ. (2004) Respiratory and haemodynamic effects of acute postoperative pain management: evidence from published data. British Journal of Anaesthesia 93: 212–23.

Cohen MR, Smetzer J. (2005) Patient-controlled analgesia safety issues. Journal of Pain and Palliative Care Pharmacotherapy 19: 45–50.

Chumbley GM, Hall GM, Salmon P. (1999) Why do patients feel positive about patient-controlled analgesia? Anaesthesia 54: 386–9.

Dolin SJ, Cashman JN, Bland JM. (2002) Effectiveness of acute postoperative pain management: I. Evidence from published data. British Journal of Anaesthesia 89: 409–23.

Hudcova J, McNicol E, Quah C et al. (2005) Patient controlled intravenous opioid analgesia versus conventional opioid analgesia for postoperative pain control; a quantitative systematic review. Acute Pain 7: 115–32.

Lehman KA. (2005) Recent developments in patient-controlled analgesia. Journal of Pain and Symptom Management. 29: S72–S89.

Macintyre PE. (2001) Safety and efficacy of patient-controlled analgesia. British Journal of Anaesthesia 87: 36–46.

Macintyre PE. (2005) Intravenous patient-controlled analgesia: one size does not fit all. Anesthesiology Clinics of North America. 23: 109–23.

Mann C, Ouro-Bang'na F, Eledjam JJ. (2005) Patient-controlled analgesia. Current Drug Targets 6: 815–19.

Mather LE, Woodhouse A. (1997) Pharmacokinetics of opioids in the context of patient controlled analgesia. Pain Reviews 4: 20–32.

Olzap G, Sarioglu R, Tuncel G et al. (2003) Preoperative emotional states in patients with breast cancer and postoperative pain. Acta Anaesthiologica Scandinavica 47: 26–9.

Sidebotham D, Dijkhuizen MRJ, Schug SA. (1997) The safety and utilization of patient-controlled analgesia. Journal of Pain and Symptom Management 14: 202–9.

Silvasti M, Rosenberg P, Seppala T et al. (1998) Comparison of analgesic efficacy of oxycodone and morphine in postoperative intravenous patient-controlled analgesia. Acta Anaesthesiologica Scandinavica 42: 576–80.

Simopoulos TT, Smith HS, Peeters-Asdourian C et al. (2002) Use of meperidine in patient-controlled analgesia and the development of a normeperidine toxic reaction. Archives of Surgery 37: 84–8.

Taylor N, Hall GM, Salmon P. (1996) Is patient-controlled analgesia controlled by the patient? Soc Sci Med 43: 1137–43.

Thomas V, Heath M, Rose D, Flory P. (1995) Psychological characteristics and the effectiveness of patient-controlled analgesia. British Journal of Anaesthesia 74: 271–6.

Vincente KJ, Kada-Bekhaled K, Hillel G et al. (2003) Programming errors contribute to death from patient-controlled analgesia: case report and estimate of probability. Canadian Journal of Anaesthesia 50: 328–32.

Viscusi ER, Reynolds L, Chung F et al. (2004) Patient-controlled transdermal fentanyl hydrochloride vs intravenous morphine pump for postoperative pain. Journal of the American Medical Association 291: 1333–41.

Walder B, Schafer M, Henzi H et al. (2001) Efficacy and safety of patient-controlled opioid analgesia for acute postoperative pain. Acta Anaesthesiologica Scandinavica 45: 795–804.

White PF. (1987) Mishaps with patient controlled analgesia. Anesthesiology 66: 81–3.

Woodhouse A, Hobbes AFT, Mather LE et al. (1996) A comparison of morphine, pethidine and fentanyl in the postsurgical patient-controlled environment. Pain 64: 115–21.

Woodhouse A, Ward ME, Mather LE. (1999) Intra-subject variability in postoperative patient-controlled analgesia (PCA): is the patient equally satisfied with morphine, pethidine and fentanyl? Pain 80: 545–53.

Appendix

An example of an acute pain management flow sheet and standard orders for patient-controlled analgesia, reproduced with permission of the Royal Adelaide Hospital, Adelaide, South Australia.

ROYAL ADELAIDE HOSPITAL

ACUTE PAIN SERVICE
PATIENT-CONTROLLED
ANALGESIA (PCA)
Standard Orders

PATIENT LABEL

Unit Record No.: _____

Surname: _____

Given Names: _____

Date of Birth: _____ Sex: _____

PCA PROGRAM ORDERS:

1. **DRUG:** ....

   * = *order in mg or microgram as appropriate*

   Place appropriate drug label here

2. **CONCENTRATION:***...**/mL**

3. **BOLUS DOSE:***

   Dose:

   .... ** = *sign and date any changes*

   .... **

   If pain not controlled:

   Bolus dose may increase to ....

   Bolus dose may increase to .... **

4. **CONTINUOUS (BACKGROUND) INFUSION:***

   .... /hr (...................... mL/hr)

   .... /hr (...................... mL/hr) **

5. **LOADING DOSE:**   0 (zero)

6. **DOSE DURATION:**   "stat"

7. **LOCKOUT:**   5 minutes

ROUTE (if other than IV): ....

GENERAL ORDERS:

1. Oxygen at *2 to 4 L/min via nasal specs or 6 to 8 L/min via mask* while orders are in effect.

2. No systemic opioids or sedatives to be given except as ordered by the APS.

3. Naloxone to be immediately available.

4. One-way anti-reflux valve to be used in IV line and an anti-syphon valve must be in-line between patient and syringe at all times.

5. *Monitoring requirements:* see overleaf.

6. Record current total dose per syringe in mg or microgram as appropriate. Reset total dose to zero when syringe changed.

7. Cease PCA if the patient becomes confused.

8. For inadequate analgesia or other problems related to the analgesia, contact the rostered APS anaesthetist.

TREATMENT OF SIDE EFFECTS:

RESPIRATORY DEPRESSION (EXCESSIVE SEDATION):

1. If sedation score = 2, reduce size of the bolus dose by half and cease any background infusion.

2. If sedation score = 3 (irrespective of respiratory rate) OR sedation score = 2 and respiratory rate ≤ 6/min, give 100 microgram NALOXONE IV stat. Repeat 2 minutely PRN up to a total of 400 microgram. Cease PCA and call the APS anaesthetist.

3. If sedation score ≥ 2 revert to hourly sedation scores until sedation score < 2 for at least 2 hours.

NAUSEA AND VOMITING:

1. Give METOCLOPRAMIDE 10mg IV 4 hourly PRN.

2. If ineffective after 15 minutes, add TROPISETRON 2 mg IV daily PRN.

3. If still ineffective after another 15 minutes, add DROPERIDOL 500 microgram IV 4 hourly PRN (250 microgram if > 70 years).

SIGNATURE OF ANAESTHETIST: .... Date: ....

(Print name ....)

Cease above orders:

Signature of anaesthetist: .... Date: .... Time: ....

APS-PATIENT CONTROLLED ANALGESIA

MR 98.2

CHAPTER 8

ROYAL ADELAIDE HOSPITAL	PATIENT LABEL
PATIENT-CONTROLLED ANALGESIA (PCA) Observations and Record of Drug Administration	Unit Record No.: _____ Surname: _____ Given Names: _____ Date of Birth: _____ Sex: _____

MONITORING REQUIREMENTS: Record HOURLY for 8 hours and then 2 HOURLY

1. PAIN SCORE   2. SEDATION SCORE   3. RESPIRATORY RATE   4. CURRENT TOTAL DOSE

Pain Score:

0 = no pain

10 = worst pain imaginable

NB: record pain scores at rest and with movement eg. coughing

Sedation Score:

0 = wide awake

1 = easy to rouse

2 = constantly drowsy, easy to rouse but cannot stay awake

3 = somnolent, difficult to rouse (severe respiratory depression)

Current total dose:

Record in mg or microgram as appropriate and not in mL. Reset total dose to zero when syringe is changed.

DRUG: **Route:**

Date/Time	Dose	Pain Scores ...... X 0 2 4 6 8 10	Sed'n Score	Resp Rate	PR	BP	Comments	Signature RN or MO

0 2 4 6 8 10

July 2006

ADVERSE DRUG REACTIONS				
Drug	Date	Details		Signature

DRUG: Route:

Date/ Time	Dose	Pain Scores .... X 0 2 4 6 8 10	Sed'n Score	Resp Rate	PR	BP	Comments	Signature RN or MO

0 2 4 6 8 10

Epidural and intrathecal analgesia

Epidural analgesia is one of the most effective methods available for the management of acute pain. When local anesthetics are used, this technique is of particular benefit for the treatment of pain associated with activity, such as coughing or walking. Combined with active postoperative and post-injury rehabilitation protocols and early enteral feeding, epidural analgesia provided by local anesthetics (with or without the addition of an opioid) may lead to a reduction in postoperative complications (particularly respiratory and cardiac) and improve patient outcome, especially in the high-risk patient. This combined rehabilitation approach has resulted in so-called 'fast-track' protocols for a number of different operations. These protocols are widely used in Europe and the USA and can significantly reduce the duration of hospital stay. However, epidural analgesia is associated with a number of uncommon but significant complications, and so the potential risks must always be weighed against possible advantages for each patient.

This form of pain relief will be initiated and managed by an anesthesiologist. If it is to be used after spinal surgery, the surgeon may place an epidural catheter at the end of the operation. Nevertheless, all medical staff must have an understanding of this form of analgesia in order to be aware of possible complications and drug interactions.

The availability of adequate and specialized care must always be considered. However, epidural and intrathecal analgesia can be safely managed on general hospital wards if the following are available:

- Appropriate patient selection criteria
- Appropriate standard orders and nursing procedure protocols
- Nursing education and accreditation programs specific to epidural and intrathecal analgesia
- Regular review of the patient by an anesthesiologist
- Availability of an anesthesiologist at all times, for consultation or management of complications or inadequate pain relief
- Agreement to delegate all responsibility for pain relief to one group of specialist medical staff (anesthesiologists), with consultation of this group by other medical personnel as required.

Anatomy

The spinal cord and brain are covered by three membranes, the meninges. The outer membrane is called the dura mater. The middle layer, the arachnoid, lies just below the dura and the two form the dural sac. The inner layer, the pia mater, adheres to the surface of the spinal cord and brain. The *epidural space* lies between the dura mater and the bone and ligaments of the spinal canal (Figure 9.1). This is only a potential space containing blood vessels, nerve roots, fat and connective tissue. Deep to the arachnoid membrane is the subarachnoid or *intrathecal space*, containing cerebrospinal fluid (CSF) and the spinal cord above the level of L1–2 and the cauda equina (the lumbar and sacral nerve roots) below L1–2. The dural sac ends at S2.

To obtain *epidural analgesia*, analgesic drugs are administered directly into the epidural space. An epidural catheter is usually placed to enable repeat doses or an infusion of the drug to be given. Epidural local anesthetic drugs gain access to nerve roots and the spinal cord by crossing the dura and subarachnoid membranes. This results in segmental anesthesia or analgesia (i.e. in a belt-like distribution of variable width, depending on the amount given). Opioids and other adjuvant analgesic drugs administered into the epidural space produce

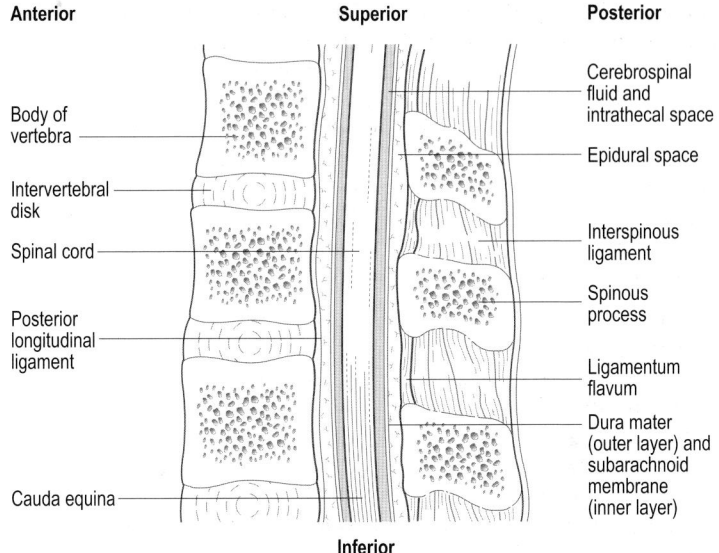

Anterior

Superior

Posterior

Body of vertebra

Intervertebral disk

Spinal cord

Posterior longitudinal ligament

Cauda equina

Cerebrospinal fluid and intrathecal space

Epidural space

Interspinous ligament

Spinous process

Ligamentum flavum

Dura mater (outer layer) and subarachnoid membrane (inner layer)

Inferior

Figure 9.1 Anatomy of the spinal cord.

analgesia via effects on the spinal cord. A proportion of the dose is also absorbed into the epidural blood vessels and enters the systemic circulation.

Drugs administered directly into the CSF and used for *intrathecal analgesia* are more commonly given as a single dose through a spinal needle at the time of spinal anesthesia. The doses of drugs required for intrathecal analgesia are much smaller than those required for epidural analgesia. Unlike epidural analgesia, intrathecal analgesia for the management of acute pain more commonly involves the administration of opioids alone, rather than a combination of local anesthetic and opioid. The opioid is delivered directly into the CSF, thereby avoiding absorption by epidural fat and blood vessels. Rostral migration in the CSF will occur, particularly with morphine. This may result in effects at higher levels of the spinal cord and even the brain.

Contraindications

The contraindications to epidural and intrathecal analgesia are summarized in Box 9.1.

Absolute or relative contraindications to epidural and intrathecal analgesia

- Untrained staff
- Patient rejection
- Contraindications to catheter or needle placement
  - local or generalized sepsis
  - large infected soft tissue injuries
  - some central or spinal neurological diseases
  - hypovolemia
  - coagulation disorders
  - concurrent treatment with anticoagulant medications
- Presence of a dural puncture

Untrained nursing and medical staff

Epidural and intrathecal analgesia should only be used in hospital wards where staff have received specific teaching about these methods of pain relief. Staff should have a good understanding of the techniques and monitoring requirements, and be able to recognize and treat (according to written orders) inadequate analgesia and side effects. Many institutions require some form of accreditation before nurses are allowed to take responsibility for patients with epidural or intrathecal analgesia. In addition, these methods of pain relief should only be used when an anesthesiologist is available to review patients at least daily and on-site, whenever problems arise.

Patient rejection

For many reasons patients may not want epidural or intrathecal analgesia. For example, they may have heard of possible complications, either from friends or from the media. A full explanation needs to be given to each patient and the risks and possible benefits explained.

Contraindications to the placement of an epidural needle or catheter

There are a number of reasons why placement of an epidural needle or catheter might be contraindicated, or at least relatively contraindicated (i.e. the potential benefits may outweigh the risks).

Infection

Epidural needles and catheters should not be placed at the site of local infection. Generalized sepsis and large infected soft tissue injuries (which could result in a bacteremia) may increase the risk of an epidural space infection, and placement of an epidural catheter in such patients remains controversial. If the patient is receiving appropriate antibiotic cover, and if the risk–benefit ratio has been considered, it may be appropriate in selected patients. The risk of performing epidural blockade in patients with human immunodeficiency virus (HIV) infection or acquired immunodeficiency syndrome (AIDS) is unknown, as is the risk of blood patch for the treatment of postdural puncture headache in these patients.

Central nervous system disease

The decision to proceed with epidural analgesia in patients with diseases such as multiple sclerosis should be made on a case-by-case basis after an assessment of risks and benefits. One of the potential issues is that any exacerbation of the disease is likely to be blamed on the analgesic technique, whereas disease progression may have been coincidental. There is no good evidence that the use of epidural techniques in these patients carries a specific risk.

Hypovolemia

The normal response to hypovolemia is peripheral vasoconstriction. If epidural local anesthetic drugs are given the resultant vasodilatation may unmask hypovolemia, leading to or contributing to hypotension. Concurrent intravenous fluids, appropriate use of vasoconstrictors and slow titration of the local anesthetic solution are recommended. The more dilute local anesthetic solutions used to provide analgesia may be less likely to contribute to hypotension.

Coagulation disorders or concurrent treatment with anticoagulant or antiplatelet medications

In general, the insertion of epidural or intrathecal needles and catheters should be avoided in patients with coagulation disorders, or in those who are fully anticoagulated. However, anticoagulant drugs may be given to patients with an epidural catheter already in place, as they are commonly prescribed for postoperative or post-trauma thromboprophylaxis. The risk of hematoma must be considered along with the potential benefits of epidural analgesia for each patient. Whenever necessary, thromboprophylaxis can be instituted after the epidural catheter has been inserted and fixed in place.

More detail about epidural analgesia and the concurrent use of anti-coagulant medications is given later in this chapter.

Presence of a dural puncture

If the dura has been punctured, either inadvertently during insertion of an epidural needle or catheter, or during spinal surgery, part of any drug injected into the epidural space may theoretically gain direct access to the CSF. The patient must be observed more closely than usual if a decision is made to proceed with epidural analgesia, although the incidence of complications arising from this may be rare.

Drugs used for epidural analgesia

Two classes of drug are commonly used for epidural analgesia: opioids and local anesthetics. They can be given as repeated bolus doses or by continuous infusion, and should be preservative free. The doses and infusion rates suggested below are guidelines only and may vary according to patient age, medical condition, site of injection and other factors.

To improve both the quality and duration of analgesia, clonidine (an α_2-adrenergic agonist) or epinephrine (adrenaline) are sometimes added to local anesthetic or opioid solutions. The epidural use of other drugs for acute pain management (e.g. neostigmine and ketamine) still requires further investigation before they can be introduced into routine clinical practice.

Regulatory approval for the epidural administration of all these drugs varies between countries, partly because the neurotoxicity studies required by some countries may not have been carried out, but also because of the varying availability of different drug preparations.

Local anesthetic drugs

Site of action

As noted earlier, epidurally administered local anesthetic drugs gain access to nerve roots and the spinal cord by crossing the dura and sub-arachnoid membranes. As with opioids and other adjuvant drugs, part of any given dose will be absorbed into the systemic circulation; use in high doses and/or over prolonged periods can carry the risk of systemic toxicity.

The level of insertion of the epidural catheter – in the middle of the dermatomal segments to be covered – is of particular importance when local anesthetics are used.

Doses

In acute pain management, combinations of local anesthetic and opioid agents are more commonly used than infusions of local anesthetic alone. There may, however, be occasions when epidural analgesia without an opioid is preferred. For example, avoidance of all opioids may be considered in a patient with severe sleep apnea, or in a patient who also requires patient-controlled analgesia (PCA) or other parenteral opioids (see below). If a local anesthetic drug is used as the sole analgesic agent, it will usually be in a concentration less than that commonly used for anesthesia (e.g. 0.0625–0.125% bupivacaine or levobupivacaine; 0.1–0.2% ropivacaine). The suggested infusion rates are similar to those prescribed for local anesthetic–opioid combinations (see Box 9.2).

Side effects

Local neurotoxicity or systemic toxicity (due to inadvertent overdose or intravascular injection) may follow epidural administration of local anesthetics (for details refer to Chapter 5). A 'total spinal', with unconsciousness and cardiovascular collapse, can occur if excessive doses are inadvertently given intrathecally.

Box 9.2

Suggestions for initial infusion rates and bolus doses using 0.0625–0.125% bupivacaine/levobupivacaine or 0.1–0.2% ropivacaine and 2–5 µ/mL fentanyl

	Younger patients (up to 40 years)	to	Older patients (over 70 years)
Infusion rate (mL/h)	8–15	to	4–12
PRN bolus doses (mL)	4–8	to	2–4

- These doses may also vary according to other factors, such as site of catheter placement and height of patient
- Thoracic epidural infusions may require slightly smaller volumes than lumbar epidural infusions
- Lower infusion rates are needed if higher concentrations of local anesthetic drugs are used
- Lower infusion rates (e.g. upper limit of 10 mL/h or less) are suggested in the elderly if the higher concentrations of opioid are used (e.g. 5µg/mL fentanyl)

Blockade of autonomic and motor fibers as well as sensory nerves may result in other side effects, including the following.

Respiratory system

The diaphragm is the most important muscle of involuntary respiration. It is supplied by cervical nerve roots 3–5, which are unlikely to be blocked by the volumes and concentrations of local anesthetic drug usually used for epidural anesthesia and analgesia. Dense motor block of intercostal muscles can reduce a patient's ability to take a deep breath and cough. However, the degree of block that occurs with the low concentrations of local anesthetic normally used for the management of acute pain is usually clinically insignificant.

Cardiovascular system

Sympathetic block can lead to hypotension. The greater the number of segments blocked and the higher the concentration and total dose of epidural local anesthetic administered, the greater the chance of hypotension.

In the low concentrations normally used in combination with opioids for pain relief on general wards, significant hypotension is unlikely unless the patient is also hypovolemic. However, even partial sympathetic blockade may prevent compensatory mechanisms from being fully effective, and may therefore unmask hypovolemia. Postural or orthostatic hypotension is also possible.

If hypotension occurs it will normally respond to intravenous fluids, but vasopressors (such as ephedrine) may be required. In some situations, and in order to avoid giving large amounts of intravenous fluids, a low-dose infusion of a vasopressor may be necessary, although this would not often be used in a general ward setting (a monitored environment is preferred). Vasopressors should be available in all wards where epidural local anesthetic agents or local anesthetic/opioid mixtures are used.

If the block extends above T4 (nipple line), and if enough local anesthetic solution has been given, the cardioaccelerator sympathetic fibers to the heart may be blocked. This can be beneficial, particularly in patients with coronary disease, and may be one reason why a high thoracic block can reduce the incidence of postoperative myocardial infarction. Any clinically significant bradycardia that occurs may respond to atropine. However, if bradycardia or hypotension is severe, titration of low doses of epinephrine (adrenaline) may be more effective.

Sedation

Unless local anesthetic doses are so large that systemic toxicity develops, they will not cause significant sedation.

Nausea and vomiting

Nausea and vomiting are much less common following epidural local anesthetics than after epidural opioids.

Pruritus

Pruritus is not a side effect of epidural local anesthetic agents.

Motor/sensory block

Immobility is not desirable after injury or surgery, so low concentrations of local anesthetic drug are used in an attempt to preferentially block smaller sensory fibers (i.e. providing analgesia) while avoiding a block of the larger motor fibers (*differential block*: see Chapter 5). Motor block and difficulty with walking are less likely to occur with thoracic epidural blockade than with lumbar placement of the catheter.

Using an infusion of low concentrations of local anesthetic drug combined with an opioid, effective analgesia can often be achieved with a minimum of motor block or block of other sensory nerves. If a patient complains of numbness or weakness, the infusion can be stopped for a short time and then restarted at a lower rate. If the problem persists, the concentration of local anesthetic may be reduced or the technique changed to use of an epidural opioid only. Numbness and weakness may also be the first signs of catheter migration into the CSF, or an epidural abscess or epidural hematoma (see later).

Patients receiving epidural infusions of a local anesthetic (or local anesthetic and opioid) can commonly sit out of bed or walk about. However, this should be done slowly and with assistance because of the risks of leg weakness, loss of position sense or postural hypotension.

Pressure areas have been reported following epidural analgesia, presumably owing to a combination of immobility and decreased sensation; appropriate pressure care should minimize this risk. Care must also be taken in patients at risk of compartment syndrome, when epidural analgesia could mask the early signs and symptoms. However, the pain that results from compartment syndrome is usually so severe that it will 'break through' the analgesia provided by low doses of local anesthetics. In some patients at risk of compartment syndrome epidural analgesia may be best avoided; if it is used, it is important to avoid motor and significant sensory blockade.

Urinary retention

As with epidural opioids urinary retention can occur, but is not inevitable and does not require routine prophylactic catheterization.

Gastrointestinal system

Bowel motility is improved by the sympathetic blockade that results from epidural administration of local anesthetic drugs. This allows for quicker recovery of gastrointestinal function after abdominal surgery and earlier enteral feeding. This benefit is more likely to be seen in patients who have thoracic epidural catheters placed for analgesia, compared with those in whom lumbar catheters are inserted.

Concerns about an increased risk of anastomotic breakdown due to increased intestinal motility appear to be unfounded; epidural analgesia using local anesthetic drugs is considered to be safe for patients undergoing bowel resection with an anastomosis. Earlier return of motility is also seen when low doses of opioids are added to the local anesthetic solution, compared with epidural opioid alone.

Opioids

Epidural opioids alone can provide good analgesia. However, most of the outcome improvements attributed to epidural analgesia are only achievable when these are combined with local anesthetics.

Site of action

Epidural and intrathecal opioids produce analgesia by blocking opioid receptors in the dorsal horn of the spinal cord. When an opioid is injected into the epidural space, some is absorbed into the epidural blood vessels and enters the systemic circulation, some binds to epidural fat, and some crosses the dura and arachnoid membranes and enters the CSF.

The proportion of epidurally administered opioid that is absorbed into the systemic circulation contributes to analgesia and to the development of opioid-related side effects. Plasma levels are highest after the administration of lipid-soluble opioids (e.g. fentanyl).

From the CSF a proportion of drug is taken up into the spinal cord. Bulk flow of CSF in a rostral direction (towards the head) means that any drug remaining in the CSF will be carried to spinal cord opioid receptors some distance from the site of injection. Rostral spread of drug has potential disadvantages, as respiratory depression may occur if sufficient opioid remains in the CSF when it reaches the brain stem and respiratory center. It can also contribute to the development of other side effects, such as nausea, vomiting and pruritus.

Differences can be seen between opioids of low and high lipid solubility when onset of effect, duration of effect (Box 9.3) and side-effect profile are compared. Less lipid-soluble drugs (e.g. morphine) take longer to cross from the epidural space to the CSF and have a slower

Box 9.3

Epidural opioids: examples of bolus doses and infusion rates

Opioid	Bolus* (mg)	Onset (min)	Peak effect (min)	Duration† (h)	Infusion* (mg/h)	Lipid solubility‡
Morphine	1–6	20–30	30–60	6–24	0.1–0.75	1
Hydromorphone	1–2	10–15	15–30	6–16	0.1–0.4	1.4
Diamorphine	2–6	5–10	10–15	6–12	0.2–1.0	280
Pethidine	20–50	5–10	15–30	1–6	10–30	39
Fentanyl	0.025–0.1	5–10	10–20	1–4	0.025–0.1	813
Sufentanil	0.01–0.05	5–10	10–15	1–6	0.01–0.05	1780

*Effective doses will vary depending on patient age, medical condition and site of injection.
†Duration of analgesia varies widely; higher doses will have a longer duration of action.
‡Octanol/pH 7.4 buffer partition coefficient.
Values may vary according to different references.

onset of action. They are cleared more slowly from the CSF, are more likely to spread rostrally, and have a longer duration of action.

The lipid-soluble drugs (e.g. fentanyl) are more rapid in onset, have a much shorter duration of action, are subject to greater vascular uptake from the epidural space, and have a more segmental spread and analgesic effect. The correct dermatomal positioning of the epidural catheter is therefore more important if lipid-soluble opioids are used.

Doses

In general, the analgesic efficacy of opioids is greater when given epidurally than with parenteral administration; that is, a smaller dose is needed in order to achieve the same or a better degree of pain relief. However, this varies according to the lipid solubility of the drug. Morphine, being the least lipid-soluble opioid used in epidural analgesia, shows the greatest difference in dose required by both routes to produce a similar analgesic effect (Box 9.4). With highly lipid-soluble drugs such as fentanyl there is little or no difference, except when very low doses are used.

Commonly used drugs, doses, approximate rate of onset and duration of action, and infusion rates are listed in Box 9.3. Because of its more rapid onset, the use of a drug such as fentanyl can be useful in the event of breakthrough pain in a patient receiving epidural morphine.

Box 9.4

Approximate equianalgesic doses of morphine according to route of administration

Oral	30 mg
Intramuscular	10 mg
Epidural	2–3 mg
Intrathecal	0.2–0.3 mg

Longer-acting opioids may be given by intermittent bolus dose or by infusion. Highly lipid-soluble opioids (e.g. fentanyl and sufentanil) are best administered by continuous infusion because of their short duration of action.

The total dose of opioid administered into the epidural space is the primary determinant of analgesic activity, but the volume in which the dose is administered may help to determine the spread of the dose. This is particularly so for more lipid-soluble opioids.

As with any opioid, the initial dose should be based on the age of the patient and subsequent doses titrated to effect. Morphine is commonly used when opioids alone are administered for epidural analgesia. Suggested initial doses given via a lumbar catheter for non-thoracic surgery or via a thoracic catheter for thoracic surgery range from 4 mg in patients less than 45 years old to 1 mg in those over 75.

Side effects

Respiratory system

Respiratory depression is a possible complication of epidural opioids.

- *Early respiratory depression* usually occurs within 2 hours of an injection (or later with an infusion) and results from high blood levels of opioid following absorption from the epidural space into the systemic circulation.
- *Delayed respiratory depression* is most commonly seen between 6 and 24 hours after the opioid was given, and results from rostral migration of drug in the CSF to the brain stem and respiratory center. The onset is usually gradual, with the patient becoming progressively more sedated. Delayed respiratory depression can persist for many hours. If naloxone is necessary it may have to be given by infusion.

Delayed respiratory depression is less likely with more lipid-soluble drugs (e.g. fentanyl and sufentanil). Once in the CSF these drugs are subject to rapid uptake into the spinal cord and blood vessels. The risk of significant concentrations of opioid reaching the respiratory center due to rostral spread is therefore much less than with morphine. However, the relatively high blood concentrations of the lipid-soluble drugs are more likely to cause early respiratory depression.

There is an increased risk of respiratory depression associated with:

• increasing patient age
• high doses of epidural (or intrathecal) opioid
• use in the opioid-naive patient
• concurrent use of sedatives or systemic opioids (including long-acting sedatives or large doses of parenteral opioid given before or during an operation).

As with other methods of opioid administration, a decrease in respiratory rate can be a late and unreliable sign of respiratory depression. Therefore, patient sedation should be frequently assessed. If a patient becomes excessively sedated, subsequent bolus doses should be reduced and infusions stopped or decreased. Naloxone may be required (see later).

Cardiovascular system

Hypotension is unlikely following epidural administration of opioids unless the patient is already hypovolemic. It has, however, been reported (rarely) following the use of pethidine (meperidine). This may be partly because pethidine has some intrinsic local anesthetic activity.

Sedation

Sedation and nausea and vomiting (see below) can occur after epidural administration of opioids. In part these side effects may result from absorption of drug into the systemic circulation; they can also be due to rostral spread of drug in the CSF.

Nausea and vomiting

It is important to remember that the cause of postoperative nausea and vomiting is often multifactorial and that conditions or drugs other than opioids may be responsible. Antiemetics should be administered and consideration given to a reduction in opioid dose. Severe and intractable nausea and vomiting may respond to opioid antagonists or agonist–antagonists (see Chapter 4).

Pruritus

Pruritus, particularly over the face, chest and abdomen, is more likely to follow epidural (and intrathecal) administration of opioids, especially morphine, than after opioids given by any other route. It appears to be less common in the older patient. Although the exact mechanism is unknown, it is presumed to be centrally mediated and a consequence of activation of μ receptors in the spinal cord. Small doses or an infusion of an opioid antagonist or agonist–antagonist can be used to treat pruritus without reversing analgesia. More recently, small doses of an anesthetic induction agent, propofol, have been noted to relieve pruritus following epidural morphine. Antihistamines may be effective in some cases, even though histamine release plays a negligible role in the development of pruritus. However, the sedative effects of these drugs may increase the risk of respiratory depression.

Other causes of itching in a hospital setting should always be considered. For example, the plastic covering of a mattress may result in sweating and itching of the back; itching may occur under dressings or plaster casts, or as an allergic reaction to antibiotics, detergents and disinfectants.

Motor/sensory block

Epidural opioids will not affect motor or sensory function.

Urinary retention

Urinary retention is a possible complication of epidural opioids and is again more likely with morphine. It is due to inhibition of the micturition reflex evoked by increases in bladder volume. However, it is not inevitable and does not require routine prophylactic catheterization of all patients. If retention does occur, small doses of an opioid antagonist or agonist–antagonist may be given. If this is unsuccessful a urinary catheter will be needed, but it can be 'in/out' and does not have to remain in situ.

Gastrointestinal system

Epidural opioids decrease bowel motility, but to a lesser degree than equianalgesic doses of opioid given by other routes.

α_2-Adrenergic receptor agonists drugs

As α receptors are a component of the descending inhibitory system of pain control within the spinal cord, the administration of an α_2 agonist has an analgesic effect. The most commonly used drugs are clonidine and epinephrine (adrenaline).

Clonidine

Neuraxial administration of clonidine has been widely investigated. There is no evidence of neurotoxicity, and it is approved for use by this route in the treatment of cancer pain by the US Food and Drug Administration.

Epidural clonidine is used mainly as an adjunct to opioids and local anesthetics. It reduces the dose of local anesthetic required for pain relief and improves the quality of analgesia. The evidence of any benefit from co-administration with opioids is weak and inconsistent.

Given in bolus doses of 25–150μg, epidural clonidine leads to both dose-dependent analgesia and dose-dependent side effects, especially sedation and hypotension. Sedation follows systemic drug absorption of the drug (the lipid solubility of clonidine is similar to that of fentanyl); hypotension occurs commonly with doses that exceed 75μg. Hypotension is likely to be greater in patients who are hypertensive or being treated for hypertension.

Epidural clonidine is not commonly used in the acute setting.

Epinephrine

Epidural epinephrine (adrenaline) has α agonist effects that lead to pain relief and also to vasoconstriction. The latter effect reduces the clearance of epidurally administered drugs, thereby increasing their duration of action. The addition of low concentrations of epinephrine to local anesthetic or local anesthetic–opioid solutions results in improved analgesia. The most commonly used concentrations are in the range of 1–2μg/mL.

Other adjuvant drugs

A number of other agents, such as ketamine and neostigmine, have been administered epidurally, primarily in experimental settings. Epidural ketamine and neostigmine, given with epidural opioids and/or local anesthetics, may improve pain relief without an increase in adverse effects. Preservative-free solutions, which should be used to avoid neurotoxicity, are not available in all countries.

Although these results are encouraging, further evaluation is needed before the use of these adjuvants becomes part of routine clinical practice.

Combinations of local anesthetics and opioids

The side effects of opioid and local anesthetic agents used in epidural analgesia are compared in Box 9.5.

In an attempt to minimize the adverse effects of each class of drug and provide better analgesia than that attained with either agent alone, a combination of low concentrations of local anesthetics and opioids in

Comparison of the possible side effects of epidural opioids and local anesthetic drugs

	Opioid	Local anesthetic
Respiratory	Delayed depression	Usually unimpaired
	Early depression	
Cardiovascular	Usually no reduction in blood pressure	Overt or postural hypotension
		Reduced heart rate with high block
Sedation	Yes	Mild/absent
Nausea/vomiting	Yes	Less common
Pruritus	Yes	No
Motor	No effect	Block
Sensation	No effect	Block
Urinary retention	Yes	Yes
Gastrointestinal	Decreased motility	Increased motility

one solution (colloquially called an 'epidural cocktail') is often used. This combination aims to promote the major outcome benefits of epidural local anesthetics and increases their analgesic efficacy; the effect appears to be synergistic. However, the amount of opioid used needs to be small in order to avoid increased adverse effects and hence reduced benefits.

Whereas the aim of the combination therapy is to obtain the full benefits of each class of drug before side effects from either class occur, the evidence for an 'optimal' concentration of each remains uncertain. Commonly used mixtures contain bupivacaine or levobupivacaine 0.0625–0.125% or ropivacaine 0.1–0.2% with 2–5 µg/mL fentanyl or 20–40 µg/mL morphine.

Other opioids that are used in combination with these local anesthetics include pethidine, diamorphine and sufentanil. It is the total dose of drugs given that is important: the higher the concentration, the lower the volume infused.

Dose regimens

Infusion rates will vary according to the concentration of drugs in the solutions, the site of injury or surgery relative to the site of epidural catheter placement, and the age of the patient. In institutions where nursing staff are allowed to administer 'top-up' doses as well as alter infusion rates, orders should include bolus doses of the solution for breakthrough pain. Suggested bolus doses and infusion rates for some of the combinations with fentanyl that may be used are listed in Box 9.2.

Requirements for the safe management of epidural analgesia

As well as the need for trained staff and the absence of contraindications to the insertion of an epidural catheter (discussed earlier), standard orders and nursing procedure protocols are recommended to maximize the safety and effectiveness of epidural analgesia. To reduce the risk of drugs or fluids intended for intravenous (IV) administration being given inadvertently via an epidural catheter, all pumps used for epidural drug administration and all epidural catheters should carry a clearly visible label; yellow is the recommended identification color. Whenever possible, only dedicated infusion pumps should be used. In addition, these pumps should ideally be rate limited (e.g. to 20 mL/h) so that large infusion rates cannot inadvertently be programmed and delivered.

Standard orders

To standardize orders throughout the institution, preprinted forms are recommended. The forms need to be completed, signed and dated by the treating anesthesiologist or pain service. An example of a preprinted epidural standard order form is provided at the end of this chapter.

It should be noted that although standard orders are used for the initial prescription of epidural analgesia, they may not be effective for all patients. At least daily evaluation by an anesthesiologist (or more often if required) will allow appropriate alterations to be made to the prescription or the analgesic technique. Daily assessment should usually include:

- Effectiveness of analgesia at rest and with activity
- Effectiveness of the treatment of any side effects
- Evaluation of any clinical features that might suggest a catheter-related complication

- An overall assessment of the patient, including the possibility of non-analgesia-related complications, and any concurrent medication orders.

Standard orders need to cover a number of different areas, as follows.

Non-drug treatment orders

Non-drug treatment orders may include a statement to eliminate the concurrent ordering of CNS depressants, other opioids and anticoagulants by other than the pain service or the responsible anesthesiologist, orders for oxygen, maintenance of IV access, and instructions on whom to contact if problems occur.

Monitoring and documentation requirements

The following should be monitored at regular intervals, the length of which might change the longer epidural analgesia continues and the more stable the patient is, but which needs to be shortened if changes in prescription or bolus doses are required:

- Pain score, sedation score and respiratory rate
- Blood pressure and heart rate
- Sensory block: block height may be measured by testing the level at which the patient reports a change in sensation from cold to warmth, e.g. when ice or alcohol is applied to the skin. However, the differences may not be very marked when low concentrations of local anesthetic drug are infused, and routine monitoring of sensory block height may not be required or possible in this circumstance. Any increasing sensory deficit should, however, be noted
- Motor block: the ability of a patient to raise a straight leg will provide evidence that lower extremity motor block is not excessive.

All observations should be documented (see the example at the end of this chapter) at regular intervals (hourly for up to 24 hours and then 2–4-hourly is suggested), along with total amount of drug delivered, dose of any drug administered for the treatment of side effects, and any changes that have been made to the infusion rates.

Drug orders

Orders for drug doses, drug concentrations, dose intervals or infusion rates, and instructions for the treatment of inadequate analgesia are required.

Orders for the treatment of side effects

The inclusion of standardized orders for the recognition and management of side effects will minimize delays in treatment.

Nursing procedure protocols

The format of nursing procedure protocols for epidural analgesia will vary with each institution, but key elements include:

- The institution's policy on accreditation (credentialing) of nursing staff
- Mechanisms for checking and discarding of opioids
- Monitoring and documentation requirements
- Instructions for:
  - administration of bolus doses
  - checking the amount of drug delivered (from the infusion pump display) against the amount remaining in the syringe/infusion bag
  - checking the infusion pump settings against the prescription (e.g. at the change of each shift)
  - checking the epidural insertion site and dressing
  - checking and documenting that the catheter is complete after removal
  - the setting up and programming of infusion pumps
  - the management of equipment faults and alarms
  - mobilization of the patient.

Patient-controlled epidural analgesia

Patient-controlled epidural analgesia (PCEA) combines the benefits of more effective analgesia with the advantages of patient control and greater patient satisfaction. Experience with PCEA for the management of acute pain is increasing with both opioids and combinations of opioid and local anesthetic drugs. Besides increased patient satisfaction, there may be a reduced need for pain service staff interventions (e.g. administration of bolus doses).

As with IV PCA, a loading dose should be given before PCEA is commenced. Unlike with IV PCA a continuous (background) infusion is more commonly ordered, although this may not always lead to better pain relief.

The parameters that have been used by some groups are listed in Box 9.6.

Box 9.6

Patient-controlled epidural analgesia: examples of parameters used

Drug	Bolus dose (mg)	Lockout interval (min)	Background infusion (mg/h)
Morphine	0.2	10	+/−0.4
Pethidine (meperidine)	10–30	5–20	+/−30
Fentanyl	0.015–0.05	5–15	+/−0.05–0.1
Sufentanil	0.004	6	+/−0.008
Hydromorphone	0.15–0.3	15–30	
Local anesthetic–opioid combinations, e.g.			
Bupivacaine 0.05–0.125% + 2–5µg/mL fentanyl	2–5 mL	10–20	+6–12 mL/h

Management of inadequate analgesia

In general, it is best to establish epidural anesthesia using stronger concentrations of local anesthetic agent before the lower-concentration local anesthetic/opioid solutions used for analgesia are commenced. The analgesic infusion should be started before the initial block has regressed completely. Continued resolution of motor and sensory blockade will usually proceed despite the infusion of a lower-concentration solution. A reduction in the intensity of motor and sensory block, as well as satisfactory analgesia, should be evident before the patient is transferred to a general ward.

If a patient complains of inadequate pain relief, initial assessment must also consider causes of pain other than that related to ineffective epidural analgesia. It is important to identify the cause, as it may not be the same pain for which epidural analgesia was first commenced. Examples include pain resulting from a postoperative complication (such as developing peritonitis or compartment syndrome, leading to pain that is severe enough to 'break through' the epidural analgesia), or pain at sites distant to the incision and related to the surgery but not covered by epidural analgesia (e.g. shoulder-tip pain following laparoscopic or thoracic surgery). Another example would be a patient with an epidural catheter placed for pain from fractured ribs but with additional painful injuries at other sites. This can be beneficial, particularly in patients with coronary disease, and may be one reason that a high thoracic block can reduce the incidence of postoperative myocardial infarction.

In some of these situations additional analgesia may be required. If other opioids are needed in addition to epidural analgesia (e.g. by PCA) it may be appropriate to use local anesthetic drugs only in the epidural infusion, so that opioids are given by one route only (in order to minimize the risk of respiratory depression).

If pain appears to be related to the surgery and better epidural analgesia is required, the procedures outlined in Box 9.7 can be tried.

Box 9.7

Management of inadequate analgesia*

Reassess the patient

- Consider another cause for new or increased pain, such as the development of postoperative or post-injury complications, e.g. bowel perforation and/or peritonitis after abdominal surgery, compartment syndrome after orthopedic surgery or limb injury, or other pain not covered by epidural analgesia
- Test for the level of the block using ice or alcohol

Bilateral block but inadequate spread (e.g. 'too low')

- Give a bolus dose of opioid or opioid/local anesthetic solution and increase the rate of an infusion

Unilateral block

- Suggests that catheter tip may have exited the epidural space through an intervertebral foramen, or that there is an anatomical reason for asymmetrical spread
- Try a larger bolus dose (anesthesiologist only) and/or withdraw catheter a few centimeters (allow adequate time after any heparin administration)

No block or generally poor pain relief

- Exclude intravascular catheter migration by aspiration test (anesthesiologist only)
- Check position of catheter using a 'test dose' of 3–8 mL of local anesthetic solution (e.g. 1% lidocaine or 0.25% bupivacaine) and test for level of sensory block ('test dose' to be administered by an anesthesiologist only)
- If 'test dose' shows no block the catheter is displaced: order alternative analgesia or reinsert catheter (allow adequate time after any heparin administration)

*These strategies are suggestions only and may not be needed in, or be suitable for, the treatment of all patients.

'Step-down' analgesia

Unlike PCA, epidural doses cannot be used as a guide for the prescription of subsequent analgesic regimens. If opioids are prescribed (parenteral or oral), appropriate age-based doses are suggested (see Chapters 4 and 7).

Patients and staff need to be aware that in view of the excellent pain relief commonly provided by epidural administration of analgesic drugs, discontinuation may be accompanied by a significant increase in pain intensity. 'Step-down' analgesia needs to be titrated in a way that can accommodate for this change in pain control. In particular, there should be some overlap of pain therapies so that the 'step-down' regimen has time to have an effect before epidural analgesia is withdrawn. Many pain services discontinue the epidural infusion but leave the catheter in situ for a while. This allows for a return to epidural analgesia should the change to systemic analgesia fail.

If the discontinuation of epidural analgesia is accompanied by change in clinical responsibility for the patient's pain management, then this change needs to be clearly understood by all staff.

Complications and side effects of epidural analgesia

Complications of epidural analgesia may be related to the epidural needle or catheter, the equipment, or side effects of the drugs (Box 9.8). The management of complications related to epidural needles or catheters is summarized in Box 9.9.

Postdural puncture headache

Whenever the dura is punctured, either intentionally or unintentionally, leakage of CSF can occur. This can lead to a decrease in CSF pressure and tension on meningeal vessels and nerves, which can result in headache. The risk of dural puncture is estimated to be about 0.16–1.3%, with the subsequent risk of headache ranging from 16% to 86%. It is less with smaller needles, certain types of needle, and in older patients.

The signs and symptoms are fairly typical and usually occur 1–2 days after the puncture. The headache is usually bifrontal and/or occipital, worse if the patient sits or strains, and may be associated with nausea and vomiting, photophobia, depression and tinnitus. Severe cases may be associated with diplopia or other cranial nerve palsies, resulting

---

Box 9.8

Possible complications of epidural analgesia

Related to the insertion of an epidural needle or catheter

- Postdural puncture headache
- Nerve or spinal cord injury
- Epidural hematoma
- Epidural space infection/meningitis
- Catheter migration

Related to the equipment

- Catheter/filter
- Infusion pumps

Related to the use of opioid and/or local anesthetic drugs

---

from traction on these nerves. Very rarely, intracranial bleeding has resulted.

Initial treatment consists of bed rest, hydration and analgesia (simple or opioid). In some centers caffeine has been used with success. If these measures are not effective a 'blood patch' can be performed. This means that another epidural needle is inserted and, in a sterile manner, 10 mL of the patient's blood are injected into the epidural space. This effectively seals the hole through which the CSF is leaking. Relief from the headache is almost immediate in 95% of cases; in case of failure it can be repeated. Blood patches may occasionally cause minor backache or headache.

Nerve or spinal cord injury

Injuries to nerves or spinal cord from needle or catheter placement are very uncommon and it is therefore difficult to obtain an exact estimate of the risk. Results from large surveys suggest that the incidence is in the range of 1 in 2000 to 1 in 20 000, although many of the cases were of a temporary nature and recovered completely with time.

In a considerable number of instances neurological problems have occurred in the presence of – but not because of – epidural analgesia. For example, paraplegia can result from a decrease in spinal cord blood flow unrelated to epidural blockade, such as hypotension due to bleeding, increased intra-abdominal pressure leading to raised epidural venous pressure, injury to an anterior spinal artery, or cross-clamping of an aorta. Damage to lumbosacral nerve roots may also occur during labor

Box 9.9

Management of complications related to epidural needles or catheters*

Dural puncture headache

- History and examination to exclude other cause of headache
- Bed rest as required for patient comfort only
- Analgesia (simple and/or opioid)
- Hydrate (oral or IV)
- Blood patch if required

Nerve or spinal cord injury

- Immediate neurological assessment
- A thorough history and examination will help to determine the site and extent of injury as well as the time of onset of signs and symptoms (the injury may be unrelated to the epidural needle or catheter)

Epidural space infection or hematoma

- Perform a history and examination (* a patient with an epidural abscess may be afebrile)
- Immediate neurosurgical assessment
- MRI scan (contrast CT if no MRI)
- Urgent surgical decompression will usually be required if neurological changes develop due to nerve or spinal cord compression, and if there are no contraindications to surgery
- Antibiotic therapy alone may be appropriate in the absence of significant neurological deficit

Epidural catheter migration

- Treat as for complications of excessive opioid and/or local anesthetic doses

Epidural catheter/filter disconnection

- If the disconnection is witnessed, it may be reasonable to clean a section of catheter with an alcohol wipe (allowing to dry completely), then cut with sterile scissors and attach a new filter

Leaking at the epidural insertion site

- If some leaking is noted at the epidural insertion site, the catheter may be left in situ if still providing adequate analgesia

*These strategies are suggestions only and may not be needed in, or suitable for, the treatment of all patients.

and delivery due to pressure from the presenting fetal part. Any signs and symptoms of spinal cord or nerve root injury require immediate neurological assessment.

Most local anesthetic drugs administered in commonly used concentrations and doses do not cause nerve damage. However, rare neurological complications have been reported after intrathecal administration of local anesthetic drugs, as outlined in Chapter 5.

Epidural hematoma

The exact incidence of epidural hematoma following epidural anesthesia or analgesia is unknown, but is estimated to be in the range of 1 in 10 000 to 1 in 100 000. Risk factors include multiple attempts at needle insertion, coagulation disorders, and concurrent administration of anticoagulants (see below). Epidural hematomas have also been reported to occur spontaneously in patients with bleeding disorders, or in those taking anticoagulant medications.

Diagnosis and treatment

The onset of signs and symptoms may be sudden. Importantly, in many patients a neurological deficit (especially muscle weakness) may be the first indication of a hematoma. Neurological dysfunction (motor, sensory, bladder or bowel) develops as the hematoma increases in size and compresses nerve roots or spinal cord. The patient may also complain of sharp back or nerve root pain. Immediately after epidural or spinal anesthesia the first signs may be an unusually dense or patchy block, or one that is unusually slow to resolve. Presentation of an epidural hematoma may be delayed for a few days after catheter insertion or removal.

Magnetic resonance imaging (MRI) is the preferred diagnostic imaging procedure and should be organized urgently in parallel with a neurosurgical consultation.

Treatment

An urgent neurosurgical consultation should be requested, as surgical decompression within 8–12 hours of the onset of neurological signs and symptoms will allow the best chance of full recovery.

Prevention

Although it may not be possible to prevent the development of a hematoma, attempts should be made to minimize the risk. In particular, as discussed later, anticoagulation or coagulation disorders must be considered in making decisions on epidural analgesia; care should be taken with the timing of insertion and removal of an epidural catheter in relation to anticoagulant administration.

It is possible, however, to maximize the chance of early detection of a hematoma, thus allowing early treatment. This requires a high index of suspicion when clinical features that might suggest a hematoma are seen, and the use of epidural analgesia in a way that does not mask the onset of neurological signs and symptoms.

Ideally, postoperative epidural analgesia should provide good pain relief with little or no motor or sensory block (this is more easily achieved with the use of thoracic catheters). This permits evaluation of the patient's neurological status throughout the period of analgesia. Nursing staff should be aware of the early signs and symptoms of a hematoma and should regularly monitor and record motor and sensory function. Any deficit should be reported immediately to the anesthesiologist or pain service concerned. If a motor or sensory deficit develops, it is almost always due to the local anesthetic agent in the epidural infusion solution, or to a cause other than an epidural hematoma. However, this should not be assumed, and any leg weakness should be presumed to indicate epidural hematoma (or abscess – see below) until proved otherwise. Temporary cessation of the infusion may be appropriate until it can be shown that these signs will resolve.

It is also important for the patient to be aware of the need to report any motor or sensory changes as well as alterations in bladder or bowel function.

Epidural space infection

Infections of the epidural space are also uncommon complications of epidural analgesia; again, the reported incidence is in the range of 1 in 2000 to 1 in 10 000. Infection may result from direct needle or catheter inoculation, infusion of contaminated fluid, hematogenous spread during episodes of bacteremia, or by tracking of a superficial infection at the site of insertion along the catheter to the epidural space. The last is probably the most common, as the majority of infections are caused by various *Staphylococcus* organisms. If an abscess develops, nerve root or spinal cord compression may result. Meningitis has also been reported.

Like epidural hematomas, epidural space infections often occur spontaneously, usually as the result of hematogenous spread of bacteria (estimated to account for up to 2 in 10 000 hospital admissions).

Diagnosis

The signs and symptoms of an epidural abscess may be similar to those of an epidural hematoma, except that onset is often later and slower. The most frequent presenting symptoms are increasing and persistent back pain, back tenderness, and signs of infection. Importantly, the patient may not be febrile. If neurological signs develop they may be delayed until some days later, although this is not always the case. Presentation of an epidural abscess may be delayed until days or weeks after the patient has been discharged from hospital.

MRI is superior to other methods of imaging and should be the diagnostic test of choice if available (with or without contrast enhancement). CT scans have given false or inconclusive findings, although reliability may be improved if contrast enhancement is used. CT scans may be used if rapid access to MRI is not possible.

Patients with meningitis may present with fever, severe headache, photophobia, neck stiffness and altered levels of consciousness. A lumbar puncture should be performed to confirm the diagnosis (but not if an abscess is suspected, as contamination of the intrathecal space may result).

Treatment

An urgent neurosurgical consultation should be requested if an abscess is suspected. In the absence of neurological complications, epidural space infections have been successfully treated with antibiotics. However, the development of any neurological changes indicates the need for an urgent neurosurgical consultation, as surgical decompression within 8–12 hours after onset of neurological signs and symptoms will allow the best chance of full recovery.

Prevention

As with an epidural hematoma, it may not be possible to prevent the development of an epidural space infection, but every attempt should be made to minimize the risk. For example, the catheter should always be inserted using an aseptic technique and epidural infusion solutions should be prepared under sterile conditions. Possible patient-related risk factors include sepsis, diabetes, depressed immune status, steroid therapy and alcohol abuse. If epidural analgesia is to be used in these patients, a risk–benefit assessment should always be carried out. Duration of catheterization is a predictor of risk, but epidural infections have been reported as soon as one day after insertion of an epidural catheter.

It is possible to maximize the chance of early detection of an abscess if epidural analgesia is used in a way that does not mask the onset of neurological changes, and if staff maintain a high index of suspicion. Should infection occur, early recognition and treatment will reduce the chance of more serious and permanent sequelae. The approach outlined above for epidural hematomas should be followed.

In addition, the catheter insertion site should be inspected daily and note taken of the patient's temperature. The catheter should usually be removed if there is inflammation or tenderness at the insertion site. Significant local infection should be treated with the appropriate antibiotics, and surgical drainage may be required. If the patient develops a fever greater than would be expected in the immediate postoperative period, consideration may be given to removal of the catheter, unless the perceived benefit of continuing outweighs possible risks.

There appears to be little benefit from routine culture of epidural catheter tips after removal, as positive cultures may be as high as 30%. This presumably results from contamination of the tip on removal of the catheter, and the results are therefore not reliable predictors of epidural space infection.

Patient education and involvement are again important. Patients must be instructed to report to the hospital or their anesthesiologist immediately if any problems are noted after discharge. An information sheet to be taken home may serve as a reminder (some examples are given at the end of Chapter 2).

Catheter migration

Rarely a catheter placed in the epidural space will migrate into the intrathecal space or an epidural blood vessel. If migration is not recognized, large doses of drugs (opioids and/or local anesthetics) intended for epidural administration will be delivered into the CSF or systemic circulation. Migration into the intrathecal space will usually result in rapidly increasing block height, whereas migration into a blood vessel leads to a loss of block and increasing pain.

Complications due to catheter migration will be more obvious and of greater magnitude if bolus doses of epidural opioid and/or local anesthetic drug are given.

Problems related to equipment

Epidural catheter or filter

Disconnection of the catheter from the epidural filter can result in contamination of the end of the catheter and migration of bacteria into the infusion solution. If this disconnection is witnessed and it is important for epidural analgesia to continue, it may be reasonable to reconnect the catheter after the outside of it has been thoroughly cleansed with an antiseptic solution and 10–20 cm trimmed from its end with sterile scissors. This should not be done without consulting the anesthesiologist responsible for the analgesia.

Kinking of the catheter can occur, making infusion or administration of a bolus dose difficult or impossible. The length of the catheter should be checked for obvious kinks; if none is visible it may be worth pulling the catheter back by 1–2 cm (time of any heparin administration allowing). Slight flexion of the patient's back may also overcome the problem.

Leaking filters should be replaced, as there is a risk of contamination of the epidural solution. If the catheter appears to be leaking at the insertion site it may be that the tip is no longer in the epidural space but lying in subcutaneous tissue. In this case, analgesia is likely to be inadequate. If pain relief appears adequate, the leakage might be due to backtracking of the infusion solution along the catheter and treatment may be continued.

The catheter should be inspected on removal to ensure that the tip is complete. If it is not, the patient should be told and details entered in their record. The catheter material is inert and surgical removal of the tip is usually unnecessary.

Infusion pumps

Operator error can lead to misprogramming of infusion pumps; pumps may malfunction; or patients may attempt to interfere with the running of the pumps. Ideally, dedicated pumps should be used.

Fatal or near-fatal doses of epidural analgesic drugs have been given when infusion pumps delivering the epidural solution have been mistakenly programmed to the rate prescribed for the infusion of intravenous fluids. A wide variety of drugs intended for intravenous administration has also been injected or infused into the epidural space. Clear labeling of all epidural catheters and infusion devices used for epidural analgesia is therefore strongly recommended. Color-coded (yellow) infusion lines and dedicated epidural pumps may help to prevent such errors, as will electronic safeguards against incorrect programming (e.g. internal upper limits for infusion rates).

Excessive doses of epidural infusion solutions have also been administered when the contents of a syringe or infusion bag have accidentally been allowed to empty by gravity. Therefore, infusion devices without antisiphon valves should be placed at an appropriate level relative to the patient.

Side effects related to the drugs

Possible side effects of epidural and intrathecal opioids and local anesthetic agents were outlined earlier in this chapter (see Box 9.5). Side effects will be exaggerated if doses intended for epidural administration are inadvertently given directly into the CSF. Suggestions for the management of these complications are listed in Box 9.10.

Care must be taken to ensure that a bolus dose of the epidural analgesic solution is not inadvertently administered during the changing of any syringes. Drug-related problems may also occur if there are errors in prescription, either by mistake or due to inadequate knowledge.

Box 9.10	
Management of side effects of epidural analgesia*	
Nausea/vomiting	Administer antiemetics and *add* additional antiemetics if ineffective
	Consider other possible causes (e.g. ileus)
	If nausea seems related to epidural analgesia, consider omitting the opioid (if used in combination with a local anesthetic) or changing to another opioid
Pruritus	Check that pruritus is likely to be related to the epidural analgesia
	Administer small doses of IV naloxone or an opioid agonist–antagonist (e.g. nalbuphine)
	?Administer an antihistamine (watch for sedation)
	If pruritus seems related to epidural analgesia, consider omitting the opioid (if used in combination with a local anesthetic) or changing to another opioid
Sedation/respiratory depression	Check no other reason for sedation (e.g. administration of a sedative)
	Sedation score 2, respiratory rate > 8/min: reduce the size of bolus doses and/or the rate of infusion
	Sedation score 2, respiratory rate < 8/min: reduce the bolus dose and/or infusion rate; consider naloxone

	Sedation score 3 (regardless of respiratory rate): administer naloxone 100 μg IV and repeat PRN
	A decrease in opioid concentration may be required, or the opioid can be omitted if being used in combination with a local anesthetic
Urinary retention	Try small doses of IV naloxone (if opioid only being used)
	Catheterize – 'in/out' or indwelling
Hypotension	Look for hypovolemia and other causes of hypotension
	Administer IV fluids +/− vasopressors as appropriate
	Cease/reduce (often only temporarily) infusion if needed (often not required)
Numbness/weakness	Check for catheter migration (into CSF)
	Cease infusion for a short time; restart at a lower rate once there is evidence of resolution of sensory and motor deficit
	Consider reducing local anesthetic concentration if above fails
	Consider urgent exclusion of spinal cord compression by hematoma/infection if there is no resolution of sensory and motor deficit within a reasonable time

* These strategies are suggestions only and may not be needed in, or be suitable for, the treatment of all patients.

Concurrent anticoagulant or antiplatelet medications

In general, insertion of epidural or intrathecal needles and catheters should be avoided in patients with coagulation disorders or in those who are fully anticoagulated. However, anticoagulant drugs may be given to patients with an epidural catheter already in place, as they are commonly prescribed for postoperative or post-trauma thromboprophylaxis.

The following recommendations are not evidence based, as the incidence of epidural hematomas is very small and therefore controlled studies are not possible. They are based primarily on expert opinion and, in particular, on consensus statements published by the American Society of Regional Anesthesia and Pain Medicine. They are not intended to provide a 'standard' of care, but to offer reasonable options for care. They cannot replace an individual risk–benefit analysis for every patient by an anesthesiologist.

Oral anticoagulants

There is little information about the risks of epidural hematoma in association with the use of warfarin. In patients on chronic warfarin therapy, hemostasis may require 4–6 days to normalize once the drug is stopped. Coagulation status should be checked before the insertion of an epidural needle or catheter; most experts would regard an INR <1.5 as safe for the insertion or removal of an epidural catheter in this setting.

Some patients are prescribed low-dose warfarin for postoperative thromboprophylaxis (e.g. after major orthopedic surgery). The best time for removal of an epidural catheter in these patients is not known. In some centers catheters are removed within 24–36 hours of the first postoperative dose. If the catheters are left in for longer than 36 hours, monitoring of coagulation status is suggested. It is of note that up to 20% of patients may show some prolongation of prothrombin time after a single dose of warfarin.

Standard unfractionated heparin (IV)

Epidural catheterization appears to be relatively safe in patients who are heparinized either during or after surgery. However, consideration must be given to the timing of both needle and catheter placement *before* heparin is given and catheter removal *after* heparin is commenced. It has been suggested that epidural needles and catheters be placed at least 1–2 hours before heparin is given. In patients likely to receive large doses of heparin (e.g. during cardiac surgery) epidural catheters are sometimes sited the day before. If a postoperative heparin infusion is required, the catheter should be removed after the infusion has been suspended for a few hours (after discussion with the treating physician). It may take 4–6 hours for activated partial thromboplastin times (APTT) to decrease to suitable levels, and measurement of the APTT before catheter removal is recommended.

Standard unfractionated heparin (subcutaneous)

Low-dose standard heparin is commonly administered for thromboprophylaxis and is generally considered safe to use in patients with concurrent epidural analgesia. However, appropriate precautions should be taken regarding the timing of catheter insertion and removal. The peak effect of a dose of standard heparin is likely to be seen at about 1 hour; duration of effect may be 4–6 hours or more.

Epidural catheters should be inserted or removed with this interval in mind. Some centers would time removal for 2 hours before the next dose in a twice-daily regimen (commonly 5000 units bd), and may omit a dose in a thrice-daily regimen. In both situations the next dose of heparin would not be given until 2 hours after removal of the catheter.

It is of note that, despite the low doses, a small number of patients will develop therapeutic plasma levels. Longer therapy with heparin can result in heparin-induced thrombocytopenia, and this may necessitate a platelet count prior to insertion or removal of an epidural catheter.

Low molecular weight heparin

In December 1997, the US Food and Drug Administration issued a public health advisory report regarding the risk of epidural hematoma in association with epidural and spinal anesthesia in patients receiving low molecular weight heparin (LMWH) as postoperative thromboprophylaxis.

Although LMWHs are used worldwide, the risk of epidural hematoma appeared to be much higher in the USA than in Europe. Reports from the USA concerned the LMWH enoxaparin, where the recommended dose after major joint replacement surgery was 30 mg twice a day. In Europe and Australasia the recommended dose is 40 mg just once a day (20 mg only may be used for some non-orthopedic and lower-risk patients). The higher risk in the USA was probably a result of higher doses and a twice-daily dosing schedule, because a trough in anticoagulant activity between doses (which may allow for safer catheter removal) is less likely to occur.

The time to peak effect of a dose of LMWH is about 3–5 hours; normal hemostasis may not return until more than 12 hours after that dose. Therefore, the timing of catheter insertion and removal must be considered carefully. These agents are excreted by the kidney, and accumulation can occur in patients with renal impairment.

The concern about the risk of epidural hematoma in association with LMWH has led to the promulgation of guidelines. It is suggested that epidural catheters should only be placed at least 12 hours after a standard prophylactic dose of LMWH. Timing of catheter removal is also important. One system is to introduce a hospital-wide policy asking for LMWH injections to be given in the evening, as removal the next morning (at least 12 hours after the last dose) allows easier monitoring of neurological function throughout the day. Another way, if LMWH is given in the mornings, is to still remove the catheter the next morning (22–24 hours after the last dose), and ask for the next dose of LMWH to be given 2 hours later.

The epidural catheter should not be removed until at least 12 hours after the last dose of LMWH and the next dose should not be given until at least 2 hours after removal.

Monitoring of all patients receiving epidural analgesia (especially those where the possibility of abnormal coagulation exists) should include immediate reporting of new pain in the back or legs, as well as any changes in neurological status.

Non-steroidal anti-inflammatory drugs and other antiplatelet agents

The use of non-steroidal anti-inflammatory drugs (NSAIDs), including aspirin (given alone), has not been identified as a risk factor for epidural hematoma. However, concurrent use with other medications that affect coagulation status may increase the risk. There is no generally accepted test that can reliably assess platelet function. Therefore, if they are required in combination with other anticoagulants, COX-2 inhibitors should be used in preference to non-selective NSAIDs.

The recommended intervals between other antiplatelet agents and the institution of neuraxial blockade are dependent on their duration of effect: 4–8 hours for eptifibatide and tirofiban, 24–48 hours for abciximab, 7 days for clopidogrel and 14 days for ticlopidine. However, these recommendations may change as clinical experience with these newer agents increases.

Thrombolytic and fibrinolytic therapy

In general, epidural analgesia should be avoided in patients receiving thrombolytic therapy (e.g. streptokinase) because of the increased risk of bleeding.

Key points

Evidence level

I All techniques of epidural analgesia for all types of surgery provide better postoperative pain relief than parenteral opioid administration

I Epidural local anesthetics improve oxygenation and reduce pulmonary infections and other pulmonary complications compared to parenteral opioids

I Thoracic epidural analgesia utilizing local anesthetics improves bowel recovery after abdominal surgery

I Thoracic epidural analgesia extended for more than 24 hours reduces the incidence of postoperative myocardial infarction

I Epidural analgesia is not associated with increased risk of anastomotic leakage after bowel surgery

II Thoracic epidural analgesia reduces incidence of pneumonia and need for ventilation in patients with multiple rib fractures

II The combination of thoracic epidural analgesia with local anesthetics and nutritional support leads to preservation of total body protein after upper abdominal surgery

II Epidural clonidine prolongs the effects of local anesthetics

II Epidural epinephrine (adrenaline) in combination with a local anesthetic improves the quality of postoperative thoracic epidural analgesia

IV The risk of permanent neurological damage in association with epidural analgesia is very low; the incidence is higher where there have been delays in diagnosing an epidural hematoma or abscess

IV Immediate decompression (within 8 hours of the onset of neurological signs) increases the likelihood of partial or good neurological recovery

IV Anticoagulation is the most important risk factor for the development of epidural hematoma after neuraxial blockade

Clinical practice points

The provision of epidural analgesia by continuous infusion or patient-controlled administration of local anesthetic-opioid mixtures is safe on general hospital wards, as long as supervised by an anesthesia-based pain service with 24-hour medical staff cover and monitored by well-trained nursing staff

Consensus statements of experts guide the timing and choice of regional anesthesia and analgesia in the context of anticoagulation, but do not represent a standard of care and will not substitute for the risk–benefit assessment of the individual patient by the individual anesthetist

Intrathecal analgesia

The contraindications, complications and the management of complications of intrathecal analgesia are similar to those for epidural analgesia. Standard orders and nursing procedure protocols are also recommended.

Drugs used for intrathecal analgesia

Opioids alone (i.e. not a combination of local anesthetic and opioid) are commonly used for intrathecal analgesia in acute pain management. The opioid is delivered directly into the CSF, avoiding absorption by epidural fat and blood vessels. Rostral migration in the CSF will occur, particularly with morphine.

In some centers, infusions of local anesthetics (sometimes combined with opioids) via intrathecal catheters at very low infusion rates (in the range of 1 mL/h of dilute solutions as for epidural infusion) are used successfully to provide postoperative analgesia. There is also increasing interest in the use of adjuvant drugs such as clonidine, dexmedetomidine (a more selective α_2-receptor agonist than clonidine) and neostigmine, although their use in the management of acute pain remains uncommon. There is currently little good evidence to show that the addition of clonidine to an intrathecal opioid is more effective than clonidine or the opioid alone.

Doses

The doses of opioids administered intrathecally are much smaller than those required for epidural analgesia. As with epidural opioid analgesia, the more lipid soluble the drug the more rapid the onset and the shorter the duration of action.

The drugs listed in Box 9.11 have all been used for intrathecal analgesia. Because pethidine (meperidine) has local anesthetic as well as opioid properties, it has been used as the sole spinal anesthetic agent (in larger doses of 30–50 mg) for a variety of lower limb operations.

Although most intrathecal opioids are given as a 'once-only' dose at the time of spinal anesthesia, a catheter may occasionally be left in place. All spinal catheters must be clearly labeled to distinguish them from epidural catheters.

Possible side effects

Side effects are similar to those that occur with epidural opioids. Although some believe that the incidence is higher with intrathecal opioids, to a large extent this is dose dependent.

If respiratory depression occurs following the administration of intrathecal morphine the time of peak risk is about 8–10 hours after injection, but can be much later. Respiratory depression appears to peak 5–20 minutes following intrathecal administration of highly lipid-soluble drugs. Increasing patient age, high doses of intrathecal opioid, an opioid-naive patient and concurrent use of sedatives or systemic opioids are associated with an increased risk of respiratory depression.

Box 9.11

Intrathecal opioids: examples of doses used

Opioid	Dose (mg)	Onset (min)	Duration (hrs)
Morphine	0.1–0.5	15–30	8–24
Pethidine (meperidine)	10–25	5–10	6–12
Fentanyl	0.006–0.05	<10	1–4
Sufentanil	0.005–0.02	<10	2–6
Diamorphine	0.5–1	<10	10–20

Management of inadequate analgesia

Usually intrathecal opioids are administered as a single dose, so that if analgesia is inadequate supplementation with oral or parenteral opioids will be required. As this may increase the risk of respiratory depression, smaller than average doses (e.g. half the normal size bolus doses for PCA) should be administered initially and increased only if they prove to be inadequate.

Key point Clinical practice point

Evidence level

I Evidence that the addition of clonidine to an intrathecal opioid is more effective than clonidine or the opioid alone is weak and inconsistent

II Intrathecal morphine at doses of 100–200 μg offers effective analgesia with a low risk of adverse effects

Clinical practice point

Clinical experience with morphine, fentanyl and sufentanil has shown no neurotoxicity with normal clinical intrathecal doses

Reproduced with permission from Acute Pain Management: Scientific Evidence ANZCA and FPM (2005).

References and further reading

Australian and New Zealand College of Anaesthetists, Faculty of Pain Medicine (ANZCA, FPM). Acute pain management: scientific evidence, 2nd edn. Melbourne: Australian and New Zealand College of Anaesthetists, 2005. Also available online at: *http://www.anzca.edu.au/publications/acutepain.htm* and *http://www7.health.gov.au/nhmrc/publications/synopses/cp104syn.htm*

Ballantyne JC, Carr DB, deFerranti S et al. (1998) The comparative effects of postoperative analgesic therapies on pulmonary outcome: cumulative meta-analyses of randomized, controlled trials. Anesthesia and Analgesia 86: 598–612.

Beattie WS, Badner NH, Choi P. (2001) Epidural analgesia reduces postoperative myocardial infarction: a meta-analysis. Anesthesia and Analgesia 93: 853–8.

Block BM, Liu SS, Rowlingson AJ et al. (2003) Efficacy of postoperative epidural analgesia: a meta-analysis. Journal of the American Medical Association 290: 2455–63.

Bonnet F, Marret E. (2005) Influence of anaesthetic and analgesic techniques on outcome after surgery. British Journal of Anaesthesia 95: 52–8.

Borgeat A, Blumenthal S. (2004) Nerve injury and regional analgesia. Current Opinion in Anaesthesiology 17: 417–21.

Bulger EM, Edwards T, Klotz P et al. (2004) Epidural analgesia improves outcome after multiple rib fractures. Surgery 136: 426–30.

Candido KD, Stevens RA. (2003) Post-dural puncture headache: pathophysiology, prevention and treatment. Best Practice and Research in Clinical Anaesthesiology 17: 451–69.

Davis DP, Wold RM, Patel RJ et al. (2004) The clinical presentation and impact of diagnostic delays on emergency department patients with spinal epidural abscess. Journal of Emergency Medicine 26: 285–91.

Grewal S, Hocking G, Wildsmith JA. (2006) Epidural abscesses. British Journal of Anaesthesia 96: 292–302.

Hebl JR, Horlocker TT, Schroeder DR. (2006) Neuraxial anesthesia and analgesia in patients with preexisting central nervous system disorders. Anesthesia and Analgesia 103: 223–8.

Horlocker TT, Wedel DJ. (2000) Neurological complications of spinal and epidural anesthesia. Regional Anesthesia and Pain Medicine 25: 83–98.

Horlocker TT, Wedel DJ, Benzon H et al. (2003) Regional anesthesia in the anticoagulated patient: defining the risks (the second ASRA Consensus Conference on Neuraxial Anesthesia and Anticoagulation). Regional Anesthesia and Pain Medicine 28: 172–97.

Holte K, Kehlet H. (2001) Epidural analgesia and risk of anastomotic leakage. Regional Anesthesia and Pain Medicine 26: 111–7.

Kehlet H. (2005) Fast-track colonic surgery: status and perspectives. Recent Results in Cancer Research 165: 8–13.

Moen V, Dahlgren N, Irestedt L. (2004) Severe neurological complications after central neuraxial blockades in Sweden 1990–1999. Anesthesiology 101: 950–9.

Niemi G, Breivik H. (2002) Epinephrine markedly improves thoracic epidural analgesia produced by a small-dose infusion of ropivacaine, fentanyl, and epinephrine after major thoracic or abdominal surgery: a randomized, double-blinded crossover study with and without epinephrine. Anesthesia and Analgesia 94: 1598–605.

Paech M. (2005). Epidural blood patch – myths and legends. Canadan Journal of Anesthesia 52: R1–5.

Rathmell JP, Lair TR, Nauman B. (2005) The role of intrathecal drugs in the treatment of acute pain. Anesthesia and Analgesia 101: S30–43.

Reihsaus E, Waldbaur H, Seeling W. (2000) Spinal epidural abscess: a meta-analysis of 915 patients. Neurosurgical Reviews 23: 175–204.

Schug SA, Pfluger E. (2003) Epidural anaesthesia and analgesia for surgery: still going strong? Current Opinion in Anaesthesiology 16: 487–92.

Schug SA, Saunders D, Kurowski et al. (2006) Neuraxial drug administration: A review of treatment options for anaesthesia and analgesia. CNS Drugs 20: (in press).

Shapiro A, Zohar E, Zaslansky R et al. (2005) The frequency and timing of respiratory depression in 1524 postoperative patients treated with systemic or neuraxial morphine. Journal of Clinical Anesthesia 17: 537–42.

Simpson RS, Macintyre PE, Shaw D. et al. (2000) Epidural catheter tip cultures: results of a 4-year audit and implications for clinical practice. Regional Anesthesia and Pain Medicine 25: 360–7.

Standl T, Burmeister MA, Ohnesorge H et al. (2003) Patient-controlled epidural analgesia reduces analgesic requirements compared to continuous epidural infusion after major abdominal surgery. Canadian Journal of Anaesthesia 50: 258–64.

Tziavrangos E, Schug SA. (2006) Regional anaesthesia and perioperative outcome. Current Opinion in Anaesthesiology 19: (in press).

Walker SM, Goudas L, Cousins MJ et al. (2002). Combination spinal analgesic chemotherapy: a systematic review. Anesthesia and Analgesia 95: 674–715.

Waurick R, Van Aken H. (2005) Update in thoracic epidural anesthesia. Best Practice and Research in Clinical Anaesthesiology 19: 201–13.

Wheatley RG, Schug SA, Watson D. (2001) Safety and efficacy of postoperative epidural analgesia. British Journal of Anaesthesia 87: 47–61.

Appendix

An example of an acute pain management flow sheet and standard orders for epidural, intrathecal and other regional analgesia, reproduced with permission of the Royal Adelaide Hospital, Adelaide, South Australia.

ROYAL ADELAIDE HOSPITAL
ACUTE PAIN SERVICE
EPIDURAL/INTRATHECAL/
REGIONAL ANALGESIA
Standard Orders

PATIENT LABEL

Unit Record No.: _____

Surname: _____

Given Names: _____

Date of Birth: _____ Sex: _____

ANALGESIA ORDERS: *(sign and date any changes)*

1. **DRUG:** ....

Place appropriate drug label here

2. **CONCENTRATION:** ....

3. **BOLUS DOSE:**

.... to .... mL 2 hourly PRN

4. **INFUSION RATE:** ** = *sign and date any changes*

.... to .... mL/hr

.... to .... mL/hr**

INTRATHECAL MORPHINE DETAILS (as needed)

Dose .... microgram

Time given ....

ROUTE: ....

GENERAL ORDERS:

1. Oxygen at *2 to 4 L/min via nasal specs or 6 to 8 L/min via mask* while orders are in effect.
2. No systemic opioids or sedatives to be given except as ordered by the APS.
3. No anticoagulant or antiplatelet medications to be given (other than heparin for prevention of DVTs) before consulting with the APS.
4. Naloxone to be immediately available.
5. An anti-syphon valve must be in-line between patient and syringe at all times.
6. Maintain IV access while orders are in effect.
7. *Monitoring requirements:* see overleaf.
8. Record current total volume per syringe in mL and reset to zero when syringe changed.
9. For inadequate analgesia or other problems related to the analgesia, contact the rostered APS anaesthetist.

TREATMENT OF SIDE EFFECTS:

RESPIRATORY DEPRESSION (EXCESSIVE SEDATION):

1. If sedation score = 2, reduce rate of infusion by one quarter to one third.
2. If sedation score = 3 (irrespective of respiratory rate) OR sedation score = 2 and respiratory rate ≤ 6/min, give 100 microgram NALOXONE IV stat. Repeat 2 minutely PRN up to a total of 400 microgram. Cease infusion and call the APS anaesthetist.
3. If sedation score ≥ 2 revert to hourly sedation scores until sedation score < 2 for at least 2 hours.

NAUSEA AND VOMITING:

1. Give METOCLOPRAMIDE 10mg IV 4 hourly PRN.
2. If ineffective after 15 minutes, add TROPISETRON 2 mg IV daily PRN.
3. If still ineffective after another 15 minutes, add DROPERIDOL 500 microgram IV 4 hourly PRN (250 microgram if > 70 years).

SEVERE ITCHING:

Give 100 microgram NALOXONE IV stat. Repeat 10 minutely PRN up to a total of 400 microgram.

SIGNATURE OF ANAESTHETIST: .... Date: ....

(Print name ....)

Cease infusion: Date: .... Time: .... **Remove analgesia catheter:** Date: .... Time: ....

Give next dose of heparin at: Date: .... Time: ....

Signature of Anaesthetist: ....

Catheter removed and complete: Signature of RN: .... Date: .... Time: ....

APS-EPIDURAL/INTRATHECAL/REGIONAL ANALGESIA **MR 98.0**

ROYAL ADELAIDE HOSPITAL	PATIENT LABEL
EPIDURAL/INTRATHECAL/ REGIONAL ANALGESIA Observations and Record of Drug Administration	Unit Record No.: _____ Surname: _____ Given Names: _____ Date of Birth: _____ Sex: _____

MONITORING REQUIREMENTS: **Record Items 1 to 6 EACH HOUR for 8 hours and then 2 HOURLY**

1. **PAIN SCORE**
2. **SEDATION SCORE**
3. **RESPIRATORY RATE**
4. **BP AND HEART RATE**
5. **MOVEMENT AND SENSATION**
6. **CURRENT TOTAL DOSE**

After administration of a <u>bolus</u> dose:
Record Items 1 to 5 every 5 minutes for 20 minutes.

After <u>removal</u> of an epidural catheter:
Record movement and sensation every 4 HOURS for 24 HOURS.

7. **EPIDURAL INSERTION SITE:** Once per shift, record any inflammation, tenderness, swelling or leakage at the epidural insertion site; reinforce dressing if needed – do not remove and replace.

Pain Score:	**Sedation Score:**
0 = no pain	0 = wide awake
10 = worst pain imaginable	1 = easy to rouse
NB: record pain scores at <u>rest</u> and <u>with movement</u> eg. coughing	2 = constantly drowsy, easy to rouse but cannot stay awake
	3 = somnolent, difficult to rouse (severe respiratory depression)

Current total dose:
Record in mL. Reset total dose to zero when syringe is changed.

Movement and Sensation:
- Ask the patient if they have any numbness/weakness. Unless injured, get the patient to flex their hips and knees (ie, draw their knees up to their chest).
- IF ALL IS NORMAL, record M✓ S✓ in the M/S column; otherwise document and call the APS immediately.

DRUG: **Route:**

Date/ Time	Dose	Pain Scores .... X 0 2 4 6 8 10	Sed'n Score	Resp Rate	PR	BP	M/S	Comments	Signature RN or MO

0 2 4 6 8 10

July 2006

ADVERSE DRUG REACTIONS				
Drug	Date	Details		Signature

DRUG: **Route:**

Date/ Time	Dose	Pain Scores .... X 0 2 4 6 8 10	Sed'n Score	Resp Rate	PR	BP	M/S	Comments	Signature RN or MO

0 2 4 6 8 10

10 Other regional and local analgesia

The use of local anesthetics for pain relief is increasingly being extended into the postoperative or post-injury period via techniques other than epidural analgesia. The growing popularity of continuous peripheral nerve blockade (CPNB) may be due to a number of factors, including concerns about the risks of epidural analgesia, especially in patients taking anticoagulant or antiplatelet medications; the ability to provide selective analgesia with minimal systemic adverse effects (which may be an advantage in some patients, such as the elderly); and the ability, in some centers at least, to send some ambulatory surgery patients home with local anesthetic analgesia.

Continuous peripheral nerve blockade

A 'single-shot' peripheral nerve block (one-time nerve or nerve plexus block) with injection of a local anesthetic agent is common practice in anesthesia. Although this may provide many hours of analgesia, an alternative technique will be required if pain relief is to be continued for a longer period. The benefits of 'single-shot' blockade can be sustained for a number of days if a catheter is placed at the time of nerve or plexus block. This allows local anesthetic drugs to be given by repeated bolus doses or by continuous infusion, and can facilitate ongoing physiotherapy and rehabilitation.

Continuous peripheral nerve blockade can often be used without the need for supplemental systemic analgesia. In general, compared with parenteral opioid analgesia, including via PCA, CPNB leads to better pain relief and fewer opioid-related side effects. In some circumstances it may even be as effective as epidural analgesia (e.g. after thoracotomy and orthopedic surgery), again with a lower incidence of side effects. In particular, techniques that avoid sympathetic blockade will be associated with a much lower incidence of hypotension.

Upper limb

A catheter placed near the brachial plexus (by any of the usual approaches, such as interscalene, supraclavicular, infraclavicular and axillary) can be used to provide pain relief after most types of upper limb surgery or injury (e.g. traumatic amputation). The infraclavicular approach allows easier and more reliable fixation of catheters to the chest wall. In addition to analgesia, the sympathetic blockade that results may be beneficial in situations where vasodilatation of blood vessels is required (e.g. after microvascular surgery, or if the patient has an ischemic arm or hand). Similarly, interscalene catheters can be used for continuous pain relief after shoulder surgery.

Lower limb

Continuous regional nerve blockade of the femoral nerve (including 'three-in-one' blocks of the femoral, obturator and lateral femoral cutaneous nerves), sciatic or posterior tibial nerves or the lumbar plexus can provide excellent analgesia following surgery or injury to the lower limb.

Catheters may also be placed adjacent to, or directly into, the sheath of a transected nerve following limb amputation (e.g. the sciatic nerve following an above-knee amputation). These are often called 'stump' catheters.

Thoracic

Similarly, continuous paravertebral blockade has been used for pain relief after thoracic surgery. It may also be as or more effective than epidural analgesia in some circumstances. Continuous intercostal or interpleural blockade has also been used, but pain relief from these techniques is probably not as good.

Analgesic drugs used with CPNB

Local anesthetics

As is the case with epidural analgesia, the aim will usually be to provide good pain relief (and possibly sympathetic blockade) without significant motor block. This allows motor function to be monitored and (where indicated) physiotherapy to be carried out. Minimal sensory block will also enable sensation to be checked and reduce the risk of pressure areas.

The degree of block produced will depend on the dose of local anesthetic drug given: the lower the total dose, the less the chance of significant motor blockade. Examples of solutions commonly used for infusion are 0.125% bupivacaine or levobupivacaine, or 0.2% ropivacaine. In case of accidental overdose or drug accumulation, levobupivacaine and ropivacaine are less cardiotoxic and there is a better responsiveness to resuscitation than with bupivacaine. Ropivacaine may also reduce the risk of long-term myotoxicity at the site of infusion, compared with bupivacaine.

In some patients, such as those with an ischemic hand or arm, a stronger concentration may be needed for adequate analgesia. The risk of a greater degree of motor block must be balanced against the need for pain relief for each patient.

Opioids

Apart from pain relief following intra-articular injection of morphine, there is no evidence that adding opioids to the solutions used for CPNB is of any benefit.

Clonidine

Clonidine is often added to local anesthetic drugs to increase the duration of 'single-shot' nerve blocks (e.g. sciatic nerve). However, there is no good evidence that it improves analgesia with CPNB.

The CPNB 'prescription'

Reported infusion and bolus dose regimens vary considerably, often according to anatomical location, and there is no good information on which to base any firm recommendations. However, in general, infusion rates of up to 8–10 mL/h of a local anesthetic such as 0.2% ropivacaine or 0.125% bupivacaine or levobupivacaine, and bolus doses of 3–5 mL, are reasonably common. Some forms of CPNB (e.g. femoral) may require the higher infusion rates and bolus doses, whereas lower rates and bolus doses may be effective with others (e.g. interscalene).

Lower infusion rates (e.g. 4–6 mL/h) of a stronger concentration of local anesthetic may be preferred for use with stump catheters, as there is a better chance of the stump dressing remaining relatively dry.

Whatever the choice of CPNB, the chance of inadequate analgesia increases if a surgical block is not properly established before the continuous infusion or bolus doses start. The initial block is usually best performed while the patient is awake, although this may not be possible in all circumstances.

Patient-controlled CPNB

Patient-controlled CPNB, using patient-controlled bolus doses with or without a continuous background infusion (which may improve pain relief), can also be used. To date, evidence for any benefit over CPNB managed by a continuous infusion alone is inconsistent. Overall, a low basal infusion rate of 3–5 mL/h with small bolus doses of 3–5 mL and a 30–60-minute lockout seems to be the preferred technique.

Although it is not yet a common technique in many centers, a number of forms of CPNB (e.g. interscalene, infraclavicular, axillary and popliteal sciatic) have been used in patients who are discharged home after surgery. However, successful and safe use of these ambulatory local anesthetic infusions requires careful patient selection, use of reliable infusion devices (reusable or disposable), good patient and carer education (including verbal and written information and 24-hour contact numbers), and appropriate patient follow-up (home visits versus phone calls).

Requirements for the safe management of CPNB

Continuous regional nerve blockade will normally be initiated and managed by anesthesiologists. Standard orders and nursing policies and procedures are recommended, and are often similar to those used for epidural analgesia (see Chapter 9). Requirements for the safe use of CPNB are also similar to those for epidural analgesia; however, the risks of severe complications are much lower (see Chapter 9).

All CPNB catheters and pumps filled with local anesthetics should be identified with a clearly visible label.

Specific care must be taken with regard to the positioning of an analgesed limb in order to avoid pressure areas and nerve compression. Patients should also be warned about the risk of decreased sensation, e.g. when using sharp tools or touching hot items.

Complications of CPNB

Complications arising from the drugs used

Local anesthetic toxicity, due either to inadvertent intravascular injection or to an excessive dose of the drug, has been reported (see Chapter 5) and can occur in association with all CPNB.

Complications arising from insertion of the needle or catheter

Significant blood loss rather than neurological deficit seems to be the main risk when CPNB is used in patients taking anticoagulant medications, although nerve damage due to bleeding has been reported. Particular care should be taken where direct pressure on a punctured vessel is not possible (e.g. lumbar plexus or infraclavicular blocks).

Nerve damage can also occur as a result of insertion of the needle or catheter during the performance of CPNB. Most nerve injury results in residual paresthesiae only, and most of these will resolve over time. However, the most devastating complication reported has been permanent cervical spinal cord damage following injection of local anesthetic into the cord during the performance of interscalene blocks under general anesthesia.

Other complications may result from local anesthetic blockade of other than the intended nerves. For example, ipsilateral phrenic nerve block and diaphragmatic paralysis may follow brachial plexus blockade, either at the time of establishment of the block or later during the treatment period. Other complications of needle insertion include pneumothorax, also following brachial plexus blockade.

Complications arising from indwelling catheters

The indwelling catheter used for CPNB carries an inherent risk of infection and the risk increases with increasing duration of use. Although the absolute risk is small, it is most likely to occur in association with a catheter inserted via an axillary approach (<2%).

Intra-articular analgesia

Intra-articular morphine is commonly used after arthroscopic surgery on the knee. This may provide reasonable pain relief for up to 24 hours, depending on the dose given.

Less commonly, intra-articular administration of local anesthetics, either as a bolus dose or by continuous infusion, has been tried after knee and shoulder surgery. However, good evidence for reliable analgesia is currently lacking.

Wound infiltration

Infiltration of a wound with a local anesthetic at the end of surgery can provide pain relief for a short time. It may be of particular benefit for pain relief after inguinal hernia surgery. However, after more major surgery a longer duration of pain relief is preferred.

Continuous wound infiltration with local anesthetics, using an infusion pump or a disposable elastomeric device, may improve pain relief after operations such as knee ligament reconstruction and shoulder surgery, but does not appear to be as effective after abdominal surgery. It is technically much easier than CPNB as the catheter is placed under direct vision by the surgeon at the conclusion of the surgery, but pain relief is not as effective.

Patient-controlled wound infusion techniques have also been used.

Topical analgesia

Topical use of local anesthetics is often forgotten in acute pain settings. As long as the recommended maximum doses of the drugs are not exceeded, it can be a very simple and safe way of providing pain relief.

One example is during dressing changes in patients with leg ulcers. The top layers of the dressing can be removed and then the remaining layers soaked with local anesthetic and left for 10–15 minutes. Additional local anesthetic can then be added in increments as the last layers of the dressing are slowly removed. Topical EMLA cream (eutectic mixture of lidocaine [lignocaine] and prilocaine) has also been used for venous ulcer debridement.

Key points

Evidence level

I Intra-articular opioids following knee arthroscopy provide analgesia for up to 24 hours

I Evidence for a clinically relevant peripheral opioid effect at non-articular sites, including perineural, is inconclusive

I Wound infiltration with long-acting local anesthetics provides effective analgesia following inguinal hernia repair, but not open cholecystectomy or hysterectomy

I CPNB analgesia, regardless of catheter location, leads to better analgesia and fewer opioid-related side effects than opioid analgesia alone (Richman et al., 2006)

I Topical EMLA cream is effective in reducing the pain associated with venous ulcer debridement

II Continuous femoral nerve blockade provides postoperative analgesia and functional recovery superior to that with IV morphine, with fewer side effects, and comparable to epidural analgesia following total knee joint replacement surgery

II Continuous perineural infusions of lignocaine (lidocaine) result in less effective analgesia and more motor block than long-acting local anaesthetic agents

II Wound infiltration with continuous infusions of local anesthetics improves analgesia and reduces opioid requirements following a range of non-abdominal surgical procedures

*Reproduced with permission from Acute Pain Management: Scientific Evidence ANZCA and FPM (2005).

References and further reading

Australian and New Zealand College of Anaesthetists, Faculty of Pain Medicine (ANZCA, FPM). Acute Pain Management: Scientific Evidence, 2nd edn. Melbourne: Australian and New Zealand College of Anaesthetists, 2005. Also available online at: *http://www.anzca.edu. au/publications/acutepain.htm* and *http://www7.health.gov.au/ nhmrc/publications/synopses/cp104syn.htm*

Capdevila X, Barthelet Y, Biboulet P et al. (1999) Effects of perioperative analgesic technique on the surgical outcome and duration of rehabilitation after major knee surgery. Anesthesiology 91: 8–15.

Capdevila X, Pirat P, Bringuier S et al. (2005) Study Group on Continuous Peripheral Nerve Blocks. Continuous peripheral nerve blocks in hospital wards after orthopedic surgery: a multicenter prospective analysis of the quality of postoperative analgesia and complications in 1,416 patients. Anesthesiology 103: 1035–45.

Davies RG, Myles PS, Graham JM. (2006) A comparison of the analgesic efficacy and side effects of paravertebral vs epidural blockade for thoracotomy – a systematic review and meta-analysis of randomized trials. British Journal of Anaesthesia 96: 418–26.

Evans H, Steele SM, Nielsen KC et al. (2005) Peripheral nerve blocks and continuous catheter techniques. Anesthesiology Clinics of North America 23: 141–62.

Horlocker TT, Kopp SL, Pagnano MW et al. (2006) Analgesia for total hip and knee arthroplasty: a multimodal pathway featuring peripheral nerve block. Journal of the American Academy of Orthopedic Surgery 14: 126–35.

Ilfeld BM, Enneking FK. (2005) Continuous peripheral nerve blocks at home: a review. Anesthesia and Analgesia 100: 1822–33.

Kalso E, Smith L, McQuay HJ et al. (2002) No pain, no gain: clinical excellence from scientific rigour – lessons learned from IA morphine. Pain 98: 269–75.

Klein SM, Evans H, Nielsen KC et al. (2005) Peripheral nerve block techniques for ambulatory surgery. Anesthesia and Analgesia 101: 1663–76.

Lee LA, Domino KB. (2005) Complications associated with peripheral nerve blocks: lessons from the ASA closed claims project. International Anesthesiology Clinics. 43: 111–18.

Leong WM, Lo WK, Chiu JW. (2002) Analgesic efficacy of continuous delivery of bupivacaine by an elastomeric balloon infuser after abdominal hysterectomy: a prospective randomised controlled trial. Australian and New Zealand Journal of Obstetrics and Gynaecology 42: 515–18.

Liu SS, Salinas FV. (2003) Continuous plexus and peripheral nerve blocks for postoperative analgesia. Anesthesia and Analgesia 96: 2638–72.

Møiniche S, Mikkelsen S, Wetterslev J et al. (1998) A systematic review of incisional local anesthesia for postoperative pain relief after abdominal operations. British Journal of Anaesthesia 81: 377–83.

Møiniche S, Mikkelsen S, Wetterslev J et al. (1999) A systematic review of intra-articular local anesthesia for postoperative pain relief after arthroscopic knee surgery. Regional Anesthesia and Pain Medicine 24: 430–7.

Navas AM, Gutierrez TV, Moreno ME. (2005) Continuous peripheral nerve blockade in lower extremity surgery. Acta Anaesthesiologica Scandanavica 49: 1048–55.

Richman JM, Liu SS, Courpas G et al. (2006) Does continuous peripheral nerve blockade provide superior pain control to opioids? A meta-analysis. Anesthesia and Analgesia 102: 248–57.

Schug SA, Jackson SA. (2005) Peripheral regional techniques for acute pain treatment. Anaesthesia and Intensive Care Medicine 6: 20–3.

Zaric D, Boysen K, Christiansen C et al. (2006) A comparison of epidural analgesia with combined continuous femoral–sciatic nerve blocks after total knee replacement. Anesthesia and Analgesia 102: 1240–6.

Zink W, Bohl JR, Hacke N et al. (2005) The long term myotoxic effects of bupivacaine and ropivacaine after continuous peripheral nerve blocks. Anesthesia and Analgesia 101: 548–54.

Non-pharmacologic therapies

Non-pharmacologic therapies (Box 11.1) can also be used in the treatment of acute pain and may be beneficial for some patients in some settings. Used alone, these strategies will usually not be effective for the treatment of moderate to severe acute pain. They should therefore be considered supplementary to the analgesic techniques described in earlier chapters.

A number of the techniques described below require time and specialized training and will not be suitable for routine use in the management of acute pain.

Psychological interventions

Psychological interventions may be grouped into information and education, relaxation and attentional strategies, cognitive behavioral interventions and hypnosis (see Box 11.1).

Information and education

Information given to patients can be:

Box 11.1

Examples of non-pharmacological therapies

Psychological	Information and education
	Relaxation and attentional strategies
	Cognitive behavioral interventions
	Hypnosis
TENS	
Acupuncture	
Physical	Immobilization
	Applications of heat or cold
	Exercise

- *procedural*: details of the planned medical or surgical treatment
- *sensory*: descriptions of the sensory experiences that a patient may expect during that treatment.

Appropriate education and information (see Chapter 2) about expected levels of discomfort, ways to decrease pain and details of all procedures may reduce distress and analgesic use and improve pain relief and clinical recovery. For some patients, however, especially those with high levels of anxiety or poor coping skills (e.g. a tendency to use denial or avoidance to deal with problems), excessive information and the need to make decisions can exacerbate distress and pain. As far as possible, the information given should therefore be tailored to each patient.

Relaxation and attentional strategies

Relaxation strategies (e.g. controlled breathing and muscle relaxation) have been used in the acute pain setting, although good evidence of benefit is lacking.

Attentional techniques include distraction (e.g. listening to music) and imagery (e.g. imagining pleasant events or scenes). These methods need not be complicated to be effective. They are easy to teach, but need periodic reinforcement. There is some evidence that these strategies may help to reduce postoperative pain.

Cognitive behavioral interventions

Cognitive behavioral therapies are derived from the study of learning and behavior change. They can be used to alter the way in which patients perceive, interpret and react to pain, and can lead to improved pain relief. These interventions may include training in coping methods or behavioral instruction, and aim to help patients understand more about their pain, take an active part in pain assessment and control, and alter their behavior in response to pain. Importantly, the patient needs to be an active participant in the process.

Hypnosis

Hypnosis has usually been used for the management of acute pain associated with medical procedures (e.g. burns care, bone marrow aspiration) and childbirth. In these settings it has been shown to provide effective pain relief.

Transcutaneous electrical nerve stimulation

Transcutaneous electrical nerve stimulation (TENS) is normally used in combination with other pain relief therapies and not as the sole means of treatment for acute pain. It may reduce analgesic requirements and subjective reports of pain after some operations and other acute pain states in some patients, if effective 'doses' (strong, subnoxious intensities) are used. The analgesic effects of TENS are thought to result, at least in part, from the release of endogenous opioids.

The technique is simple, safe, non-invasive, free from systemic side effects, and allows patients some control over their own therapy. The battery-powered TENS unit generates a small electric current which is transmitted to electrodes placed on the skin. The best effect is achieved when the electrodes are placed over the affected dermatomes or over acupuncture points, although trials of different combinations of electrode positions as well as TENS settings may be needed. The amplitude and frequency of the current delivered are varied by the patient according to the severity of the pain. The current is altered so that it is intense enough only to produce a comfortable buzzing or tingling on the skin. Both high-frequency (e.g. 100 Hz) and low-frequency (e.g. 2–4 Hz) currents have been used with TENS. It is possible that better results are obtained by using a mixed mode (i.e. an alternating pattern of high and low frequencies). The duration and pattern of TENS may also alter its effectiveness. Intermittent stimulation (e.g. for 30 minutes at a time) may be better than prolonged or continuous stimulation.

It is suggested that TENS not be used over a pregnant uterus unless the patient is in labor, and that it should be avoided in patients with cardiac pacemakers and implanted defibrillators. Electrical interference may disrupt normal cardiac pacemaker function – 'demand' pacemakers may sense the stimulus from the TENS unit as cardiac activity. Stimulation over the anterior neck may result in laryngospasm or hypotension.

Skin irritation may occur at electrode sites but is rarely serious.

Acupuncture

Acupuncture may be effective in the treatment of acute pain in a number of different settings (e.g. in labor or after surgery), when it can reduce pain intensity and opioid consumption. It has also been used effectively in the prevention and treatment of nausea and vomiting.

Physical interventions

Applications of heat or cold, massage, exercise and immobilization (e.g. of a limb) may help to relieve pain and muscle spasm, especially that associated with back and other musculoskeletal injuries.

Key points

Evidence level

I Combined sensory–procedural information is effective in reducing pain and distress

I Training in coping methods or behavioral instruction prior to surgery reduces pain, negative affect and analgesic use

I Certain stimulation patterns of TENS may be effective in some acute pain settings

I Acupuncture may be effective in some acute pain settings

II Hypnosis and attentional techniques reduce procedure-related pain

Reproduced with permission from Acute Pain Management: Scientific Evidence ANZCA and FPM (2005).

References and further reading

Australian and New Zealand College of Anaesthetists, Faculty of Pain Medicine (ANZCA, FPM). Acute Pain Management: Scientific Evidence, 2nd edn. Melbourne: Australian and New Zealand College of Anaesthetists, 2005. Also available online at: *http://www.anzca.edu.au/ publications/acutepain.htm* and *http://www7.health.gov.au/ nhmrc/publications/synopses/cp104syn.htm*

Bjordal JM, Johnson MI, Ljunggreen AE. (2003) Transcutaneous electrical nerve stimulation (TENS) can reduce postoperative analgesic consumption. A meta-analysis with assessment of optimal treatment parameters for postoperative pain. European Journal of Pain 7: 181–8.

Carroll D, Tramèr M, McQuay H et al. (1997) Transcutaneous electrical nerve stimulation in labour pain: a systematic review. British Journal of Obstetrics and Gynaecology 104: 169–75.

Chernyak GV, Sessler DI. (2005) Perioperative acupuncture and related techniques. Anesthesiology 102: 1031–49.

Cyna AM, McAuliffe GL, Andrew M. (2004) Hypnosis for pain relief in labour and childbirth: a systematic review. British Journal of Anaesthesia 93: 505–11.

Johnston M, Vogele C. (1993) Benefits of psychological preparation for surgery: a meta analysis. Annals of Behavioral Medicine 15: 245–56.

Lynch L, Simpson KH. (2002) Transcutaneous electrical nerve stimulation and acute pain. British Journal of Anaesthesia: CEPD Reviews. 2: 49–52.

Smith CA, Collins CT, Cyna AM et al. (2003) Complementary and alternative therapies for pain management in labour. The Cochrane Database of Systematic Reviews. Issue 2. Art. No.: CD003521. DOI: 10.1002/14651858.CD003521.

Suls J, Wan CK. (1989) Effects of sensory and procedural information on coping with stressful medical procedures and pain. A meta analysis. Journal of Consulting and Clinical Psychology 57: 372–9.

Acute neuropathic and persistent postacute pain

12

Although many chronic pain states are the consequence of neuropathic pain, its role in the acute pain setting is much less well recognized. In this setting there are a small number of patients in whom neuropathic pain predominates, or contributes to the pain they are experiencing. It is often underdiagnosed and therefore undertreated.

It is important for those who look after patients with acute pain to be aware of the signs and symptoms of neuropathic pain (the time of onset of which may vary from immediately after the initial injury until quite some time later) and to be aware of the available treatment options. These patients may present with pain that is responding poorly to opioids. Some patients may be labeled as inappropriately sensitive to pain, or even as 'drug seeking', when they are simply seeking effective pain relief.

In addition, there will be some patients who, because of the type of surgery or the nature of injury sustained, are at risk of developing persistent (chronic) pain, which is also often neuropathic in origin. The incidence and severity of persistent postacute pain is widely underestimated. Early recognition and aggressive management of pain in these patients (possibly including preventive treatment – see later) may reduce the incidence and severity of subsequent persistent pain problems.

The provision of effective pain relief in these patients can be a difficult and challenging task and one that may be ongoing for weeks, months, or even years. It is recommended that advice be obtained from specialist pain medicine physicians. Often these patients need appropriate referral to chronic pain clinics for follow-up after treatment of the acute situation and discharge from hospital. Losing these patients to follow-up can delay appropriate ongoing treatment and thereby delay or impair functional recovery after otherwise successful surgery or treatment of injury.

Pathophysiology of neuropathic pain

Pain can be broadly classified into two main types, nociceptive and neuropathic (see Chapter 3).

Nociceptive pain is the most common type seen in acute clinical care and its treatment is therefore the primary focus of this book. Neuropathic pain is pain associated with injury or disease of the peripheral or central nervous system (CNS). It is also referred to as *neurogenic pain, deafferentation pain, neuralgia, neuralgic pain* and *nerve pain*. It is the pathophysiological consequence of a number of changes in the peripheral and central nervous systems that occur after nerve injury (see Box 12.1).

At a peripheral level, nerve injury leads to structural and functional changes in the damaged neuron. Alterations in ion channels (in particular sodium channels), and receptor density (e.g. of α_1 and opioid receptors) and activity, reduce the threshold for activation of the injured afferent neurons, resulting in the phenomenon of ectopic discharge. Other peripheral changes are microneuroanatomical, with axonal sprouting and cross-connectivity between efferent sympathetic fibers and nociceptors, as well as phenotypical changes in neighboring afferents (i.e. touch fibers become pain fibers).

At a central level, central sensitization develops as a result of neuroplasticity. Neuroplasticity refers to alterations that occur in synaptic processing in the CNS as a result of neuronal activity. Some of these changes underlie processes such as learning and memory. Others can lead to maladaptive or pathological states – for example the excessive excitatory response of spinal dorsal horn neurons that follows intense noxious peripheral stimuli (e.g. from surgery or injury) and leads to pain hypersensitivity or amplification of pain (central sensitization). Other central changes include the loss of large fiber inhibition and deafferentation hyperactivity. There is also increasing recognition of the role of reorganization of the somatosensory cortex as a contributing factor to

Box 12.1

Pathophysiological changes underlying neuropathic pain

Peripheral nervous system

- Ectopic discharge
  - spontaneous
  - evoked
- Microneuroanatomical changes
  - axonal sprouting
  - cross-connections
  - sympathetic-sensory coupling
- Phenotypical changes
  - touch fibers develop pain fiber behavior

Spinal cord

- Central sensitization
- Loss of large fiber inhibition
- Deafferentation hyperactivity
- Anatomical reorganization
- Reactive changes by glial cells

Brain

- Reorganization of somatosensory cortex

neuropathic pain states such as phantom limb pain and complex regional pain syndrome (CRPS).

Clinical features of neuropathic pain

The diagnosis of neuropathic pain can usually be made on the basis of a complete history and physical examination (see Chapter 3). Features that suggest neuropathic pain are listed in Box 3.1. It is important to note that not all of these have to be present in order for a diagnosis of neuropathic pain to be made.

Patients will typically describe their pain as different from 'normal' wound pain and as a 'strange' pain. The diagnosis is easy when the pain occurs in an area of neurological deficit, e.g. below the level of the lesion after spinal cord injury, or in a flaccid arm after brachial plexus injury. However, neuropathic pain can be the consequence of very minor nerve injury which does not result in any other neurological signs or symptoms and might even go undetected by diagnostic tests such as nerve conduction studies.

Acute neuropathic pain syndromes

A few of the many possible causes of neuropathic pain in the acute clinical setting are listed in Box 12.2.

Box 12.2

Examples of neuropathic pain in the acute pain setting

Postoperative

- Post-amputation
- Post-thoracotomy
- Post-mastectomy

Post injury

- Sciatica
- Spinal cord injury
- Post amputation
- Burns injury
- Brachial plexus avulsion
- Sacral root injury in association with a fractured pelvis
- Major crush injuries of upper or lower limbs

Associated with cancer

- Pancreatic cancer (involvement of the celiac plexus)
- Compression or infiltration of the brachial plexus after spread of lung cancer to apical lymph nodes
- Involvement of sacral nerve roots by pelvic lymph node metastases
- Compression or infiltration of the spinal cord by epidural metastases (impending acute danger of paraplegia)

Associated with medical illnesses

- Viral infections, e.g. acute herpes zoster (shingles)/postherpetic neuralgia, HIV/AIDS
- Post-stroke pain
- Guillain–Barré syndrome
- Diabetic neuropathy
- Alcoholic neuropathy
- Demyelinating diseases such as multiple sclerosis

Causally it makes sense to separate postoperative and post-traumatic neuropathic pain (i.e. the majority of cases presenting in an acute pain setting) from neuropathic pain caused by cancer or associated with medical illnesses. Whereas the latter two are more commonly chronic pain states, they can present acutely – for example rapidly increasing spinal cord compression by an epidural metastasis, acute herpes zoster (shingles), or Guillain–Barré syndrome.

The diagnosis of acute neuropathic pain after injury or surgery, followed by its appropriate treatment, will result in improved pain relief and patient satisfaction. Typical examples of clinical situations where acute neuropathic pain is common are burns pain, pain after a pelvic fracture that involves injury to a sacral nerve root (often accompanied by radicular pain i.e. neuropathic pain in the distribution of the injured nerve), and phantom pain after amputation.

Examples of some specific acute neuropathic pain syndromes are discussed below:

- Post-amputation pain
- Complex regional pain syndrome
  and in Chapter 13:
- Pain after burns
- Pain after spinal cord injury
- Pain associated with acute herpes zoster and Guillain–Barré syndrome.

Post-amputation pain syndromes

Amputation of a limb by trauma or surgery is inevitably associated with nerve injury. This can lead to a number of phenomena: stump pain, phantom sensations and phantom pain.

Stump pain refers to pain in the stump itself and can be nociceptive or neuropathic in origin. It is most common in the early postoperative period, usually as nociceptive wound pain. If it becomes persistent, it can lead to severe disability and interfere with the wearing of a prosthesis.

Phantom sensation is defined as any sensory perception of the missing body part with the exclusion of pain. Such sensations are experienced by almost all patients who have undergone amputation. The sensation can range from a vague awareness of the limb (possibly with associated paresthesiae) to complete sensation, including size, shape, position, temperature and movement. Although there is no treatment for phantom sensations, it is important to explain to patients that they usually diminish in intensity and size over time. 'Telescoping' of the phantom limb is a common experience: the limb gradually shrinks proximally to approach the stump.

Phantom limb pain is defined as any noxious sensory phenomenon of the missing limb and is estimated to occur in up to 85% of patients. The pain is independent of gender, cause (elective or traumatic amputation), or side of amputation, but appears to have a lower incidence in children and congenital amputees. The pain usually occurs in the distal portion of the missing limb and may resemble any preamputation pain in character and localization. Often the limb is described as being in a hyperextended or otherwise unnatural position. Phantom pain can develop immediately after amputation or have a delayed onset; in 75% of patients it occurs within the first few days.

The risk of phantom pain appears to be increased if severe pain existed prior to amputation. Other potential risk factors are severe postoperative stump pain and chemotherapy.

Phantom pain and sensations can also follow other surgery, e.g. mastectomy, excision of the tongue or rectum, or after removal of teeth.

Complex regional pain syndrome

Complex regional pain syndrome (CRPS) is another manifestation of neuropathic pain and is associated with abnormalities of the sympathetic nervous system. By definition, CRPS occurs after an inciting event (i.e. an injury or disease) that might only be minor: a fracture of the radius is one of the more common causes. The duration and severity of the pain following this inciting event exceeds the expected recovery period. In parallel, clinical features of CRPS develop, including spontaneous and/or burning pain, allodynia and hyperalgesia; changes in sensory function (decreased sensation in a quadrant or hemibody distribution); changes in motor function (reduction in motor range and strength, tremor, dystonia); and sympathetic nervous system changes (alterations in skin blood flow and temperature, edema, excessive sweating, and atrophy of skin, hair and nails).

The nomenclature differentiates between CRPS types 1 and 2. Type 1 (previously referred to as 'reflex sympathetic dystrophy' or RSD) shows the features listed above in the absence of detectable nerve injury. The term CRPS type 2 (previously referred to as 'causalgia') is used when these features occur subsequent to nerve injury.

Key point

Evidence level

IV Acute neuropathic pain occurs after surgery and trauma

Reproduced with permission from Acute Pain Management: Scientific Evidence ANZCA and FPM (2005).

Early detection and immediate appropriate treatment are the key factors to success and require acute pain therapists to be aware of these syndromes.

Treatment of acute neuropathic pain

Treatment of neuropathic pain may require a combination of pharmacologic, physical and behavioral therapies. In the acute stage, it usually begins with drug therapy (see Chapter 6 and Box 12.3) and/or the use of regional neural (neuraxial or peripheral nerve) blockade.

Pharmacological treatments

Neuropathic pain is still often regarded as unresponsive to opioids, but this is not true. Numerous studies have shown some opioid responsiveness in a number of neuropathic pain conditions. However, neuropathic pain is typically less responsive to opioids than nociceptive pain. One of the early signs of the development of neuropathic pain in the acute situation

---

Box 12.3

Pharmacological options for the treatment of acute neuropathic pain

Drugs	Examples
Opioids*	Tramadol, methadone, oxycodone, morphine
Tricyclic antidepressants	Amitriptyline, nortriptyline, imipramine, dothiepin, doxepin (venlafaxine, an SNRI, may also be effective)
NMDA receptor antagonists	Ketamine
Anticonvulsants	Gabapentinoids (gabapentin, pregabalin), clonazepam, sodium valproate, carbamazepine
Membrane stabilizers	Lidocaine (lignocaine), mexiletine
α_2-Adrenergic agonists	Clonidine
Calcitonin	
Topical agents	Lidocaine patch, capsaicin, EMLA cream

*Neuropathic pain is often only partially responsive to opioids.

---

is ineffective pain relief despite increasing doses of opioid, and possibly the onset of sedation in a patient who still reports high pain scores.

Effective analgesia is often difficult to achieve and may require the use of a number of different drugs. These are often added in a stepwise manner as needed at intervals of a few days, so that the effectiveness of each addition can be seen.

Most studies that look at the treatment of neuropathic pain investigate the management of chronic neuropathic pain states (e.g. diabetic neuropathy, postherpetic neuralgia). There is much less evidence for the treatment of acute neuropathic pain, and so management strategies must be extrapolated from evidence based on treatment of the chronic pain state.

The choice of a first-line agent depends on the criteria used for effective treatment – pain relief alone, or pain relief and quality of life (including adverse effects). If pain relief alone is chosen, current evidence suggests that tricyclic antidepressants (TCAs) are the first choice of treatment, followed in order by opioids, tramadol, and then the gabapentinoids (gabapentin and pregabalin). If pain relief and quality of life measures are the criteria for efficacy, gabapentinoids become the first-choice agent followed by tramadol, opioids and TCAs. The sequence of treatments used will inevitably be altered in clinical practice owing to factors such as clinical experience in the acute pain setting, interpatient variations, and financial constraints, as the gabapentinoids are relatively expensive.

In the acute setting, ketamine, lidocaine and clonazepam may also be useful treatment options, as may one of the older anticonvulsants (e.g. sodium valproate, carbamazepine).

For more details on the various pharmacological options, see Chapter 6.

Topical treatments

Topical agents may be useful for localized neuropathic pain states such as postherpetic neuralgia (PHN) and nerve entrapment syndromes, in particular when allodynia is a prominent feature of the pain.

In a number of countries, including the USA, lidocaine is now available as a patch for topical use. These 10 × 14 cm adhesive patches, which are very soft and contain 700 mg lidocaine, are worn over the painful area. Owing to the poor diffusion of lidocaine through the skin, they have no local anesthetic effect on the skin and no systemic effect (plasma concentrations are barely measurable). Where available, lidocaine patches are regarded as the first-line treatment of focal neuropathies, including PHN, especially in the elderly patient.

Some patients with a localized neuropathy use EMLA cream for similar purposes, but this mixture is easily absorbed systemically and the high prilocaine content can result in methemoglobinemia if used repeatedly in higher doses.

Capsaicin (the active ingredient of hot chilli peppers) is another compound used topically in these situations. It is available as a cream that is applied to the painful area several times a day. Its analgesic effect is believed to result from the depletion of substance P (a neurotransmitter) in unmyelinated sensory nerves, which then leads to a block of these nerves. When applied to the skin, capsaicin first induces a burning feeling and hyperalgesia, which is why patients sometimes like to use EMLA cream before first using capsaicin.

Topical applications of aspirin or other NSAIDs in chloroform or ether suspension have also been reported to be of some benefit.

Regional neural blockade

A variety of regional and sympathetic blocks may be of use in the treatment of neuropathic pain. For example, epidural analgesia may prevent or reduce neuropathic pain following lower limb amputation (see below); a celiac plexus block might be useful in the treatment of pain due to pancreatic cancer; stellate ganglion blocks may help otherwise intractable angina pain or the sympathetically maintained pain component in the management of CRPS of the arm; and continuous brachial plexus blockade may be used following upper limb amputation.

Transcutaneous electrical nerve stimulation

Transcutaneous electrical nerve stimulation (TENS; see Chapter 11) can also be useful, especially if stimulation of the nerve trunk proximal to the site of injury is possible.

Treatment of specific acute neuropathic pain syndromes

In general, acute neuropathic pain resulting from most causes, including the syndromes listed above, can be managed as already described. Some specific comments regarding neuropathic pain resulting from spinal cord injury, burns injury, acute herpes zoster and Guillain–Barré syndrome are made in Chapter 13, and more details outlining the management of post-amputation pain syndromes follow.

Post-amputation pain syndromes

The treatment of stump pain requires the use of multimodal analgesia for the nociceptive wound pain. However, if stump pain does not respond to this approach, then ketamine and possibly systemic lidocaine (lignocaine) may be useful.

Treatment options for phantom limb pain include those mentioned above for the management of acute neuropathic pain in general. However, it can also be treated more specifically by the use of repeated daily intravenous (IV) infusions or subcutaneous (SC) injections of salmon calcitonin (100–200 IU), after prophylactic use of an antiemetic. The institution of preventive analgesia prior to amputation (see below) is also worthwhile.

Key points

Evidence level

I There is little evidence from randomized controlled trials to guide specific treatment of post-amputation pain syndromes

II Calcitonin, morphine, ketamine, gabapentin reduce phantom limb pain

II Ketamine and lidocaine (lignocaine) reduce stump pain

Reproduced with permission from Acute Pain Management: Scientific Evidence ANZCA and FPM (2005).

Progression of acute to persistent pain

The progression of acute pain to persistent pain after surgery, trauma or acute medical disease (such as shingles) is an underestimated problem that has significant long-term consequences for the patient, as well as for health-care costs and society. One entity alone, chronic post-surgical pain (CPSP,) accounts for 20% of admissions to pain clinics, and the estimated number of new cases in the USA lies in the range of 100 000–200 000 per year.

Most of these pain states have an element of neuropathic pain. The risk of postoperative neuropathic pain appears to be higher after some operations than others, and this may lead to CPSP (see Box 12.4). Two commonly quoted examples are thoracotomy and mastectomy, where respectively an intercostal nerve or the intercostobrachial nerve may be damaged. Other operations with a high incidence of CPSP include amputation, cholecystectomy and herniotomy. Apart from the type of surgery (most likely linked to risk of nerve damage), other predictive factors for

Box 12.4

Incidence of chronic post-surgical pain

Surgery	Incidence (%)*
Limb amputation	
phantom pain	30–85
stump pain	5–62
Thoracotomy	
lateral approach	11–80
video-assisted	1–63
Breast surgery	
chest/breast/scar pain	11–57
arm/shoulder pain	12–59
phantom pain	13–24
Cholecystectomy	
open	10–48
laparoscopic	3–58
Inguinal hernia	0–63

* Reported incidences vary between studies.

CPSP have been identified. Preoperatively these include the duration and intensity of pain before surgery, psychosocial factors (psychological vulnerability, compensation), pretreatment with opioids, female gender, younger age, radiotherapy to the area of surgery, and chemotherapy.

Postoperatively, the severity of acute pain seems to be the most important predictor – an opportunity to use preventive analgesic techniques (see below). Again, psychosocial factors also play a role (e.g. depression, vulnerability, anxiety and neuroticism).

The pathophysiology of this progression process is closely linked to central sensitization (discussed earlier). This is confirmed by the finding that the extent of wound hyperalgesia in the days following surgery correlates with the incidence of CPSP. It is currently thought that hyperalgesia is a common process after tissue injury, possibly helping to encourage rest of the affected body part, but that it is also usually self-limiting. The development of persistent pain may be a maladaptive version of this normal physiological response. Last, but not least, there is increasing evidence for the contribution of reorganization and remapping of the somatosensory cortex following nerve injury, e.g. in the development of phantom limb pain and CRPS. Underlying contributing factors to the development of these changes might be genetic and/or psychosocial predisposition.

Preventive analgesia

In view of the importance of the progression of acute to chronic pain states, there has been increasing interest in strategies aimed at reducing the incidence and severity of such syndromes.

The initial concepts focused on the provision of *pre-emptive* analgesia. Studies compared the effects of administering pain-relieving drugs or techniques prior to an intervention (e.g. surgical incision) with the same drug or technique given after the intervention. This concept was based on findings in animal studies that supported the concept of pre-emptive analgesia, but it has never been convincingly demonstrated in human studies. The reasons for this are many, but most important is that this concept ignores the processes of postoperative inflammation and peripheral sensitization that continue to produce pain after surgery, and which will not be covered by the single interventions used in pre-emptive analgesic approaches.

Current interest is focusing on *preventive* analgesic strategies, where the analgesic effects exceed the expected duration of effect of the strategy. These may be started preoperatively and aim to provide analgesia throughout the postoperative period.

As activation of the NMDA receptor is a crucial component of central sensitization, it is not surprising that NMDA receptor antagonists, in particular ketamine, have been of particular interest. Ketamine has been shown to have preventive analgesic effects in some circumstances.

Another preventive option includes the early use of calcitonin. Early use of amitriptyline in acute herpetic pain may reduce the incidence of post-herpetic neuralgia.

The perioperative use of continuous regional anesthesia and analgesia may also be effective in reducing the incidence of CPSP after some operations. After lower limb amputation, epidural analgesia has been shown to reduce the incidence of severe phantom limb pain; there is little evidence for the benefit or otherwise of leg blocks, although they provide excellent postoperative analgesia; and sciatic nerve sheath catheters (or 'stump' catheter) also give good pain relief, although they have not been shown to reduce the incident of phantom pain. It is also possible that epidural analgesia will have a preventive effect if used during and after thoracotomy and abdominal surgery.

Changes in surgical approach and avoiding repeat or unnecessary surgery may also be beneficial. Techniques that are minimally invasive or minimize nerve damage may reduce the risk of CPSP.

In patients thought to be at risk of neuropathic pain after surgery or injury, it may be worth initiating therapy *before* any clinical features of neuropathic pain develop (see examples below).

Example 1

A 20-year-old patient is admitted following traumatic below-elbow amputation of an arm after an industrial accident. He is taken to the operating room for debridement of that arm.

An example of a preventive regimen that might be used for such a patient is:

- A continuous brachial plexus block using a local anesthetic infusion placed before surgery if possible and continued for 4–6 days, or morphine by patient-controlled analgesia (the former is preferable)
- An intravenous (IV) ketamine infusion at 100–200 mg/day, started during surgery and continued for 5–7 days
- Amitriptyline 25 mg at night (even if neuropathic pain does not develop while the patient is in hospital, it may be worth continuing this for 3 months based on data from other settings).

Example 2

A 60-year-old patient is scheduled for an above-knee amputation. An example of a preventive analgesic regimen that might be used for such a patient is:

- Regional analgesia, e.g. epidural analgesia or leg block (a stump catheter – that is, a catheter placed by the surgeon in or close to the sciatic nerve sheath – may also be placed after a leg block or spinal anesthesia)

- Opioid analgesia as required; regular paracetamol
- An intravenous (IV) ketamine infusion at 50–100 mg/day, started during surgery and continued for 5–7 days
- Amitriptyline 10 mg at night (even if neuropathic pain does not develop while the patient is in hospital, it may be worth continuing this for 3 months based on data from other settings).

Key points

Evidence level

I The timing of a single analgesic intervention (preincisional versus postincisional), defined as pre-emptive analgesia, does not have a clinically significant effect on postoperative pain relief

I There is evidence that some analgesic interventions have an effect on postoperative pain and/or analgesic consumption that exceeds the expected duration of action of the drug, defined as preventive analgesia

I NMDA receptor antagonist drugs in particular show preventive analgesic effects

II Some specific early analgesic interventions reduce the incidence of chronic pain after surgery

III Perioperative epidural analgesia reduces the incidence of severe phantom limb pain

Clinical practice point

Perioperative ketamine may prevent phantom limb pain

Reproduced with permission from Acute Pain Management: Scientific Evidence ANZCA and FPM (2005).

References and further reading

Australian and New Zealand College of Anaesthetists, Faculty of Pain Medicine (ANZCA, FPM). Acute Pain Management: Scientific Evidence, 2nd edn. Melbourne: Australian and New Zealand College of Anaesthetists, 2005. Also available online at: *http://www.anzca.edu.au/ publications/acutepain.htm* and *http://www7.health.gov.au/ nhmrc/publications/synopses/cp104syn.htm*

Bouhassira D, Attal N, Alchaar H et al. (2005) Comparison of pain syndromes associated with nervous or somatic lesions and development of a new neuropathic pain diagnostic questionnaire (DN4). Pain 114: 29–36.

Brennan TJ, Kehlet H. (2005) Preventive analgesia to reduce wound hyperalgesia and persistent postsurgical pain: not an easy path. Anesthesiology 103: 681–3.

Duhmke RM, Cornblath DD, Hollingshead JR. (2004) Tramadol for neuropathic pain. Cochrane Database of Systematic Reviews, CD003726.

Finnerup NB, Otto M, McQuay H et al. (2005) Algorithm for neuropathic pain treatment: an evidence based proposal. Pain 118: 289–305.

Gilron I, Bailey JM, Tu D et al. (2005) Morphine, gabapentin, or their combination for neuropathic pain. New England Journal of Medicine 352: 1324–34.

Gottschalk A, Cohen S, Yang S et al. (2006) Preventing and treating pain after thoracic surgery. Anesthesiology 104: 594–600.

Hayes C, Molloy AR. (1997) Neuropathic pain in the postoperative period. International Anesthesiology Clinics 35: 67–91.

Janig W, Baron R. (2003) Complex regional pain syndrome: mystery explained? Lancet Neurology 2: 687–97.

Katz J. (2003) Timing of treatment and preemptive analgesia. In: Rowbotham DJ, Macintyre PE, eds. Clinical pain management: acute pain. London: Arnold.

Kehlet H, Jensen TS, Woolf CJ. (2006) Persistent postsurgical pain: risk factors and prevention. Lancet 367: 1618–25.

Kvarnstrom A, Karlsten R, Quiding H et al. (2003) The effectiveness of intravenous ketamine and lidocaine on peripheral neuropathic pain. Acta Anaesthesiologica Scandinavica 47: 868–77.

McCartney CJ, Sinha A, Katz J. (2004) A qualitative systematic review of the role of N-methyl-D-aspartate receptor antagonists in preventive analgesia. Anesthesia and Analgesia 98: 1385–400.

Namaka M, Gramlich CR, Ruhlen D et al. (2004) A treatment algorithm for neuropathic pain. Clinical Therapeutics 26: 951–79.

Nicholson BD. (2004) Evaluation and treatment of central pain syndromes. Neurology 62: S30–6.

Perkins FM, Kehlet H. (2000) Chronic pain as an outcome of surgery. A review of predictive factors. Anesthesiology 93: 1123–33.

Schug SA. (2002) Is neuropathic pain an acute problem? Acute Pain 4: 43.

Shipton EA, Tait B. (2005) Flagging the pain: preventing the burden of chronic pain by identifying and treating risk factors in acute pain. European Journal of Anaesthesiology 22: 405–12.

Visser EJ. (2006) Chronic post-surgical pain: Epidemiology and clinical implications for acute pain management. Acute Pain 8: 72–81.

13 Non-surgical acute pain

Many of the significant advances in the management of acute pain in recent years have arisen from work that has focused on pain relief after surgery. Although there are obviously many other sources of acute pain, the general principles of management that have resulted from this work remain the same, regardless of the cause of the pain. The aim of this chapter is to touch briefly on some of the causes of non-surgical acute pain and some of the problems specific to acute pain management in these patients.

Burns injury

Patients suffering from burns often have a number of different reasons for their pain. Not only are they likely to have variable degrees of constant background pain and incident pain, for example when moving or coughing, but they are also repeatedly subjected to multiple, often prolonged, procedures such as dressing changes, and regular physiotherapy over a long period. Effective management of these different aspects of pain may require different treatment strategies. In addition, the pain may be a mixture of nociceptive and neuropathic, and there is a reasonably high chance of chronic pain developing.

Effective analgesia often involves both pharmacological and non-pharmacological therapies, and this is especially true in this group of patients.

Pharmacological

In the initial stages after a burns injury, pain management using intravenous (IV) opioids is usually required, unless the burns are relatively minor. In patients who are hypovolemic the absorption of intermittent subcutaneous (SC) or intramuscular (IM) injections of opioid may be delayed and unreliable. Parenteral opioid administration may be continued once the patient is comfortable, for example using patient-controlled analgesia (PCA); for less severe pain, oral opioid analgesia may suffice.

Routine administration of non-steroidal anti-inflammatory drugs (NSAIDs) may not be appropriate, either in the initial stages if the patient is hypovolemic, or in the later stages, when they could increase the risk of bleeding during surgery. COX-2 inhibitors may be suitable, as they lack any effect on platelets and might also reduce the risk of stress-induced gastrointestinal ulcers, which are not uncommon in this group of patients.

Opioids remain an important component of analgesia during procedures such as dressings. If IV PCA is prescribed, some patients may benefit from the use of an opioid with a faster onset of action than morphine (e.g. fentanyl). It is not uncommon for higher bolus doses to be required during this time, so that the patient can more easily match their opioid requirement with the inevitable increase in pain stimulus. Patients should be observed closely after the procedure ends, as opioid-related sedation and respiratory depression may follow the decrease in pain stimulus. This may be more likely if sedatives (e.g. midazolam or lorazepam) have also been given during the procedure. Anxiolytics are, however, often a necessary adjunct in these patients because of significant psychosocial stressors and anxiety.

Intranasal fentanyl may be useful in patients who do not require IV access, as the rate of onset can be almost as quick as with IV fentanyl (see Chapter 7). However, the doses required are often unexpectedly high. If oral or SC/IM opioids are given prior to an intervention such as a dressing change, sufficient time (e.g. 45–60 min) should be allowed for them to work before proceeding.

Nitrous oxide is commonly used for pain relief during burns dressings and can be very effective in selected patients, but care should be taken to minimize the risks of nitrous oxide toxicity, in particular with repeated use over longer periods (see Chapter 6).

Ketamine (also see Chapter 6), given either as a low-dose infusion or as intermittent bolus doses, is also a frequently used adjunct, especially during dressing changes. In some centers it is combined with midazolam and given as small doses (e.g. 10 mg ketamine/0.5 mg midazolam) every 3–5 minutes as needed, administered by nursing staff or by PCA.

A variety of regional analgesic techniques may sometimes be used, although in patients with more severe burns concerns about infection or bleeding, and the need to provide good pain relief for many days if not weeks, may preclude their use.

Analgesia in the later stages of a burn injury may be provided by controlled-release (slow-release) oral opioids, with additional access to immediate-release oral opioids for breakthrough and incident pain (e.g. associated with physiotherapy or minor dressing changes).

Neuropathic pain is not uncommon after burns injury, in both the early and the later stages of the treatment and recovery phases. If it does not respond well to opioids, alternative medications such as parenteral ketamine or lidocaine (lignocaine) in the early stages, and tricyclic antidepressants or anticonvulsants (e.g. carbamazepine, sodium valproate, gabapentin, pregabalin) in the later stages may be required (see Chapter 6).

Non-pharmacological

Immediately after the injury, simple procedures such as cooling and covering the burn, and immobilization of injured limbs, will help with pain relief. Other techniques that have been used, especially in the treatment of procedural pain, include hypnosis, distraction and other stress-reducing strategies (see Chapter 11).

Key points

Evidence level

IV Opioids, particularly via PCA, are effective in burns pain, including procedural pain

Clinical practice points

Acute pain following burns injury can be nociceptive
and/or neuropathic in nature, and may be constant (background pain), intermittent or procedure related

Acute pain following burns injury requires aggressive multimodal and multidisciplinary treatment

Reproduced with permission from Acute Pain Management: Scientific Evidence ANZCA and FPM (2005).

Spinal cord injury

Acute pain resulting from spinal cord injury can also be a mix of nociceptive pain (at the site of injury from musculoskeletal damage) and neuropathic pain. Neuropathic pain, at or below the level of the injury, may be reported early after the injury, or later in the recovery and rehabilitation stages.

The neuropathic pain may be localized to the level of the lesion and then radiate to the dermatomal distribution of the affected levels. In addition, patients can experience poorly localized pain below the level of the lesion, i.e. in an area of complete deafferentiation. These are often called 'phantom pains' and can be accompanied by sensation of deafferentiated body parts.

Neuropathic pain can also be a presenting symptom of impending spinal cord or nerve root injury. For example, allodynia and hyperalgesia as well as back pain may be early presenting symptoms of a developing epidural abscess (not necessarily related to epidural analgesia) or epidural metastasis, before any motor or sensory deficit occurs. If there is no neurological deficit antibiotic therapy alone may be appropriate for the treatment of an abscess, and high-dose steroids and radiotherapy for a metastasis. If the patient has signs of spinal cord compression, urgent surgical decompression is usually the treatment of choice, unless contraindicated by the patient's condition or other medical reasons.

Treatment of pain from spinal cord injury often involves the use of opioids (including tramadol) and 'simple' analgesics as well as drugs used to manage other neuropathic pain states (e.g. ketamine, gabapentin, pregabalin, lidocaine and tricyclic antidepressants). Ketamine or lidocaine (lignocaine) infusions may be the most appropriate treatment in early acute stages.

Key points

Evidence level

II IV opioids, ketamine and lidocaine (lignocaine) reduce acute spinal cord injury pain

II Gabapentin is effective in the treatment of acute spinal cord injury pain

Clinical practice point

Treatment of acute spinal cord pain is largely based on evidence from studies of other neuropathic and nociceptive pain syndromes

Specific medical conditions

Renal and biliary colic

A common misconception has been that pethidine (meperidine) is the preferred opioid for the management of renal or biliary colic. There is, however, no evidence to support this.

The initial treatment of choice for renal colic is NSAIDs, which provide better pain relief than opioids with a lower incidence of vomiting, although in some patients opioids may also be required. The onset of action will be faster if the NSAIDs are given intravenously. Anticholinergic antispasmodic drugs (e.g. hyoscine) are less effective than NSAIDs.

Parenteral NSAIDs are at least as effective as opioids for the relief of pain from biliary colic, and again are more effective than anticholinergic drugs.

Key points

Evidence level

I   NSAIDs are superior to parenteral opioids in the treatment of renal colic

I   The onset of analgesia is faster when NSAIDs are given IV for the treatment of renal colic

II There is no difference between pethidine (meperidine) and morphine in the treatment of renal colic

II Parenteral NSAIDs are as effective as parenteral opioids in the treatment of biliary colic

Reproduced with permission from Acute Pain Management: Scientific Evidence ANZCA and FPM (2005).

Acute herpes zoster

Acute herpes zoster (AHZ) infection ('shingles') is common, particularly in patients over 50 years old. Reactivation of the latent varicella zoster virus (i.e. the virus that causes chickenpox) leads to severe acute neuropathic pain in dermatomes supplied by the involved (spinal) dorsal root or cranial nerve ganglia. A painful vesicular rash also forms. A chronic form of neuropathic pain called postherpetic neuralgia (PHN) can follow – in elderly patients the incidence is up to 75%.

Analgesic agents used for both nociceptive and neuropathic pain may be needed. Topical aspirin may also be effective. In particular, the early use (within 72 hours of onset of AHZ) of antiviral agents and amitriptyline started at the time of onset of the rash and continued for a few months, may reduce the duration of acute pain and the risk of a patient developing PHN. Epidural analgesia and sympathetic blockade may also be effective for the treatment of pain from AHZ and reduce the incidence of PHN.

Combined with an antiviral agent, corticosteroids can be used systemically or topically and may reduce the acute pain and accelerate healing of the skin lesions.

Key points

Evidence level

I Antiviral agents started within 72 hours of onset of rash accelerate acute pain resolution and may reduce severity and duration of postherpetic neuralgia

II Amitriptyline use in low doses from the onset of rash for 90 days reduces incidence of postherpetic neuralgia

Reproduced with permission from Acute Pain Management: Scientific Evidence ANZCA and FPM (2005).

Sickle cell disease and hemophilia

Both these hematological diseases are inherited disorders and can lead to recurrent severe acute pain.

In sickle cell disease, vaso-occlusion of the microcirculation results in tissue ischemia and infarction. Severe pain may be reported in the back, legs, chest and arms, and pain from involvement of abdominal organs may mimic an acute abdomen. Although hypoxia can precipitate a sickle cell crisis, oxygen supplementation during a crisis does not seem to help the pain.

In patients with hemophilia, bleeding into joints and muscle is common, although other sites (e.g. the abdomen) may also be involved. These patients often use Factor VIII to reduce the pain associated with a bleed, and unless the pain is severe they may not require admission to hospital.

As with any severe acute pain, IV loading with opioids should precede the maintenance opioid regimen such as PCA or oral opioids; SC or IM injections are best avoided in patients with hemophilia. Although all opioids would be effective, the use of pethidine (meperidine) is discouraged. Some of these patients may be taking opioids long term (i.e. they are opioid tolerant – see Chapter14) and can require higher than 'usual' doses.

The inevitable and recurrent nature of the pain can have significant psychological and social consequences for these patients and multidisciplinary pain management may be needed.

Key points

Evidence level

II IV opioid loading optimizes analgesia in the early stages of an acute sickle cell crisis. Effective analgesia may be continued with intravenous (including PCA) opioids such as morphine, but pethidine (meperidine) should be avoided

II Oxygen supplementation during a sickle cell crisis does not reduce pain

Reproduced with permission from Acute Pain Management: Scientific Evidence ANZCA and FPM (2005).

Neurological disease

Pain associated with some neurological diseases, for example multiple sclerosis, Guillain–Barré syndrome, following a stroke, or associated with a peripheral neuropathy (e.g. diabetic neuropathy) is usually neuropathic in nature, although nociceptive pain (e.g. musculoskeletal) may also be present.

Guillain–Barré syndrome is usually thought of as a primarily motor neuron disease, which often leads to respiratory failure requiring ventilation. However, many patients describe severe widespread neuropathic pain, often without the features of a peripheral neuropathy, as well as musculoskeletal pain. As in these patients the pain is often severe and acute, treatment with systemic lidocaine (lignocaine) and/or ketamine as well as gabapentin and carbamazepine is often required.

A painful peripheral neuropathy may also develop in patients with HIV/AIDS, in addition to pain from a multitude of other causes. There is the possibility of complex interactions between drugs used for analgesia and those prescribed for the treatment of HIV/AIDS. Analgesic strategies will include those already previously described for the management of neuropathic pain.

Key points

Clinical practice points

Treatment of acute pain associated with neurological disorders is largely based on evidence from trials for the treatment of a variety of chronic neuropathic pain states

Neuropathic pain is common in patients with HIV/AIDS

In the absence of specific evidence, the treatment of pain in patients with HIV/AIDS should be based on similar principles to those for the management of cancer and chronic pain

Interaction between antiretroviral and antibiotic medications and opioids should be considered in this population

References and further reading

Alper BS, Lewis PR. (2000) Does treatment of acute herpes zoster prevent or shorten postherpetic neuralgia? Journal of Family Practice 49: 255–64.

Australian and New Zealand College of Anaesthetists, Faculty of Pain Medicine (ANZCA, FPM). Acute Pain Management: Scientific Evidence, 2nd edn. Melbourne: Australian and New Zealand College of Anaesthetists, 2005. Also available online at: *http: //www.anzca.edu.au/publications/acutepain.htm* and *http://www7.health.gov.au/ nhmrc/publications/synopses/cp104syn.htm*

Bowsher D. (1997) The effects of pre-emptive treatment of postherpetic neuralgia with amitriptyline: A randomised, double-blind, placebo-controlled trial. Journal of Pain and Symptom Management 13: 327–31.

Finnerup NB, Otto M, McQuay HJ et al. (2005) Algorithm for neuropathic pain treatment: an evidence based proposal. Pain 118: 289–305.

Frenay MC, Faymonville ME, Devlieger S et al. (2001) Psychological approaches during dressing changes of burned patients: a prospective randomised study comparing hypnosis against stress reducing strategy. Burns 27: 793–9.

Gallagher G, Rae CP, Kinsella J. (2000) Treatment of pain in severe burns. American Journal of Clinical Dermatology 1: 329–35.

Jung BF, Johnson RW, Griffin DR et al. (2004) Risk factors for postherpetic neuralgia in patients with herpes zoster. Neurology 62: 1545–51.

Kinsella J, Rae CP. (2003) Burns. In: Rowbotham DJ, Macintyre PE, eds. Clinical pain management: acute pain. London: Arnold.

Kumar V, Krone K, Mathieu A. (2004) Neuraxial and sympathetic blocks in herpes zoster and postherpetic neuralgia: an appraisal for current evidence. Regional Anesthesia and Pain Medicine 29: 454–61.

Moulin DE, Hagen N, Feasby TE et al. (1997) Pain in Guillain–Barré syndrome. Neurology 48: 328–31.

O'Connor A, Schug SA, Cardwell H. (2000) A comparison of the efficacy and safety of morphine and pethidine for suspected renal colic in the emergency setting. Journal of Accident and Emergency Medicine 17: 261–4.

Osterberg A, Boivie J, Thuomas KA. (2005) Central pain in multiple sclerosis – prevalence and clinical characteristics. European Journal of Pain 9: 531–42.

Rees DC, Olujohungbe AD, Parker NE et al. (2003) Guidelines for the management of the acute painful crisis in sickle cell disease. British Journal of Haematology 120: 744–52.

Siddall PJ. (2006) Pain following spinal cord injury. In: McMahon SB, Koltzenburg M, eds. Wall and Melzack's textbook of pain. Amsterdam: Elsevier.

Siddall PJ, Middleton JW. (2006) A proposed algorithm for the management of pain following spinal cord injury. Spinal Cord 44: 67–77.

More complex patients

The general principles of acute pain management apply to most patients in most acute pain settings. However, there are some groups of patients in whom effective and safe management of pain can be a little more complex. The aim of this chapter is to touch briefly on some of these groups, highlighting where concerns may arise and some possible changes that might be required in acute pain treatment regimens.

Elderly patients

Advances in anesthesia and surgery, combined with the increasing proportion of elderly people in the populations of most countries, mean that greater numbers of older patients are now presenting for major operations or after major injuries. These patients are at higher risk of complications due to unrelieved or undertreated acute pain (see Chapter 1). They are therefore particularly likely to benefit from effective pain relief. However, a number of factors may combine to make control of pain more difficult than in the younger patient. These include:

- Age-related alterations in pharmacokinetics (how the individual deals with the drug) and pharmacodynamics (how the individual responds to the drug)
- Altered perception of pain and potential difficulties in assessment
- Diminished physiological reserves and concurrent diseases
- Concurrent medications, leading to an increased risk of drug interactions.

Changes in pharmacokinetics and pharmacodynamics

Pharmacokinetics

The pharmacokinetics (absorption, distribution, metabolism and excretion) of many drugs are altered in the elderly. This is due primarily to two factors: the progressive physiological decline that occurs with increasing age, and the increasing likelihood of concurrent disease.

The physiological changes associated with aging are progressive, but the rate of decline can be highly variable between individuals (i.e. physiological aging may or may not parallel chronological aging). It is also difficult to separate changes due to age and those that result from the higher incidence of degenerative and other diseases that is inevitable in this age group. The physiological changes associated with aging that are of most significance to pharmacokinetics are related to cardiac output and renal function, although changes in liver function and protein binding may also have some effect. For a summary of the more important physiological changes and their possible effect on analgesic drug regimens see Box 14.1.

Concurrent diseases and concurrent use of other drugs may also alter these factors. For example, congestive cardiac failure and chronic liver disease may be associated with reductions in hepatic blood flow.

Pharmacodynamics

Age-related changes in pharmacodynamics also occur, although the mechanisms behind these changes are not yet fully understood. It appears that the sensitivity of the brain to opioids is increased by about 50% in the elderly. However, it is not clear whether this difference is due to alterations in the number and/or function of opioid receptors in the central nervous system, or to other factors.

Assessment of pain

The assessment of pain and evaluation of pain relief therapies may be more difficult in the elderly owing to differences in pain perception and reporting of pain, cognitive impairment, and difficulties in measurement.

Box 14.1

Key age-related physiological changes and possible effects on analgesic therapy

Parameter	Change	Effect
Cardiac output	↓ up to 20%	Increase in peak concentration after an IV bolus dose means smaller bolus doses may be needed or the dose should be given more slowly
Renal function	30% ↓ nephron mass	Smaller maintenance doses of drugs that are cleared by the kidney, or have active metabolites that are cleared by the kidney, will be needed
	10%/decade ↓ renal blood flow	
	30–50% ↓ glomerular filtration rate	The elderly should be considered to be renally impaired even if blood creatinine levels are within the 'normal' laboratory range
	50–70% ↓ creatinine clearance	
Liver function	25–40% ↓ liver blood flow	Smaller maintenance doses of some drugs that depend on the liver for metabolism (e.g. most opioids) may be required
	25% ↓ phase I enzymes	Liver enzymes responsible for demethylation decline rapidly with aging (may slow clearance of drugs such as diazepam)
Protein binding	↓ Plasma protein levels	May alter the free ('active') fraction of a drug (e.g. ↓ albumin concentrations in the elderly are associated with reduced dose requirements for diazepam)

Data from Macintyre et al. (2003).

Perception of pain

Pain thresholds and pain tolerance change in the elderly; thresholds to experimental pain are generally increased. Although the significance of these results in the clinical setting remains uncertain, they could indicate some deterioration in the early warning function of pain.

There are a number of clinical reports suggesting that some older patients may report no pain or less pain in conditions that are normally associated with severe pain. For example, 'silent' myocardial infarction is more common in the older patient; pain is less likely to be a presenting symptom in older patients with significant abdominal pathology such as peritonitis; and the elderly report less postoperative pain or pain after some procedures.

Studies looking at age-related changes in pain tolerance are more limited but show that tolerance is reduced in elderly people, meaning that severe pain could have a greater impact. Pain that is reported needs treatment as in the younger patient, especially as the development of persistent pain and/or any interference with acute rehabilitation may affect the older patient to a much greater extent.

Reporting of pain

Many factors may lead to under-reporting of pain in elderly patients. These include psychological and cultural factors such as fear, anxiety, depression, cognitive impairment, the implication of the disease, loss of independence, feelings of isolation, the quality of social support available, and family. Elderly patients, in particular those with multiple other health complaints, often tend to under-report pain to avoid being labeled as complainers. The elderly and their carers may even see pain as a normal part of aging.

Cognitive impairment

Cognitive function declines with age, and patients who have cognitive impairment are known to be at greater risk of undertreatment of acute pain, perhaps partly due to under-reporting. The reasons for this are not clear, but it could result from factors such as memory impairment, diminished pain perception, or diminished capacity to report pain. There is also a tendency among staff and carers to disbelieve the pain complaints of confused patients.

Confusion (or delirium) is a form of acute cognitive impairment. It is reasonably common in the elderly patient during acute illnesses or in the postoperative period, leading to increased morbidity and hospital stay. Although the exact cause may be unknown, a number of risk factors have been identified (Box 14.2). If a patient becomes confused while taking opioids, a common reaction is to stop the opioid. However, as confusion may be the result of many other factors (including pain itself), consideration should be given to simply reducing the dose rather than complete avoidance of the drug.

Measurement of pain

Accurate and repeated assessments of pain are necessary for effective pain management. As with younger patients, the elderly patient's self-report is the most reliable indicator of pain.

Box 14.2

Risk factors for the development of delirium

- Old age
- Pre-existing dementia
- Anticholinergic drugs (including some antiemetics), psychoactive drugs, benzodiazepines, opioids
- Withdrawal from alcohol or sedatives
- Infection
- Fluid and electrolyte imbalance
- Hypoxemia
- Severe pain
- Multiple concurrent medical problems
- Multiple concurrent medications

Measures of pain in common use in the acute setting, such as the visual analog scale (VAS), verbal numerical rating scale (VNRS) and verbal descriptor scale (VDS) (see Chapter 3), have all been used for assessment of pain in the elderly. The latter two, VNRS and VDS, are probably more reliable to use in this age group.

Patients with mild to moderate cognitive impairment may be able to understand and use the VDS but might need more time to think about and respond to questions, and repeated questioning may be required. These patients are often able to assess pain reliably at the time when asked (present pain), but recall (e.g. if asked about pain over the last few days or weeks) may be less reliable. In patients with more severe cognitive impairment, tools that can be used to assess pain include the Pain Assessment in Advanced Dementia (PAINAD) and the Abbey Pain Scale.

In non-communicative patients assessment of pain can be more difficult. Commonly, behaviors such as restlessness, tense muscles, frowning or grimacing, and grunting or groaning are used to assess pain severity. However, whereas these behaviors may be a reasonable indicator of the presence of pain, they do not necessarily indicate the severity of that pain. In addition, there may be other reasons for distress and such behaviors.

Observation of function, such as the ability to take deep breaths and cough, as well as tolerate physiotherapy and walking, is also important and may help to assess adequacy of analgesia.

Analgesic drugs

As with younger patients, a range of analgesic drugs may be used in the management of acute nociceptive and neuropathic pain. These drugs are covered in more detail in previous chapters. The comments that follow relate primarily to differences in their use or effects in the elderly.

In general, adverse effects of drugs are more common in the elderly. They include drug–drug, disease–drug and adverse drug reactions.

Opioids and tramadol

If opioids are to be used effectively yet safely in the elderly a number of factors must be considered.

Choice of drug

Pure opioid agonists are usually the drugs of choice in the elderly. Drugs with a short half-life (e.g. oxycodone) are preferred, as this facilitates rapid titration of dose. Agonist–antagonist opioids (e.g. butorphanol and nalbuphine) are generally not recommended because of a higher incidence of delirium with their use.

Accumulation of active metabolites may occur as a result of impaired renal function and decreased renal clearance. An increase in morphine 6-glucuronide levels may necessitate unexpectedly low maintenance doses of morphine, owing to its analgesic activity. Unless large doses of morphine or hydromorphone are required, problems due to the accumulation of morphine 3-glucuronide or hydromorphone 3-glucuronide (see Chapter 4) are unlikely to be seen in the acute pain setting. Pethidine (meperidine) is probably best avoided in the elderly because significant accumulation of the active metabolite, norpethidine, may occur. Accumulation of nordextropropoxyphene may lead to confusion or cardiac toxicity in the older patient. In patients with renal impairment a drug without active metabolites, such as fentanyl, may be a useful alternative.

The elimination half-life of tramadol is known to be slightly prolonged in the elderly and the active metabolite, *O*-desmethyl-tramadol (commonly known as M1), is also dependent on the kidney for excretion. Therefore, lower daily doses of tramadol may be required in the older patient.

Opioid dose and dose intervals

Opioid requirements decrease with increasing patient age. The reasons for this have not been fully explained, as noted in Chapter 4. Although total daily opioid doses are likely to be less than those needed by younger patients, the elderly will still exhibit the wide interpatient variability in opioid dose and in blood levels required for effective analgesia.

Although the effective duration of a single dose may be increased in the elderly, in the absence of any contraindication these patients should not be denied further doses solely because duration of action is expected to be prolonged.

Side effects of opioids

RESPIRATORY DEPRESSION The fear of causing respiratory depression in the elderly often leads to inadequate doses of opioid being given. As with other patients, significant respiratory depression can generally be avoided if appropriate monitoring is in place.

The elderly are at particular risk of hypoxemia in the postoperative period, and this will most often be due to factors other than opioid-induced respiratory depression, such as pre-existing disease, the surgery itself, and the respiratory effects of opioids (see Chapters 3 and 4). The elderly patient is also likely to be at higher risk from the possible adverse effects of hypoxemia, such as myocardial ischemia and infarction, cognitive impairment and confusion. In addition, as outlined above, retention of active metabolites can increase the risk of respiratory depression in elderly patients, especially those with renal impairment.

NAUSEA, VOMITING AND PRURITUS The incidence of postoperative nausea and vomiting decreases with increasing age. Routine administration of antiemetics is not recommended, as some of these drugs (particularly those with anticholinergic properties) are more likely to cause side effects in the elderly.

Pruritus appears to be less common in the elderly.

COGNITIVE EFFECTS Compared to morphine, fentanyl may cause less postoperative confusion and less change in cognitive function.

Other analgesic drugs

Changes in treatment regimens may also be required for a number of the other drugs used to manage acute pain in the older patient. Possible changes are summarized in Box 14.3.

Specific analgesic techniques

Patient-controlled analgesia

Patient-controlled analgesia (PCA) should not be withheld from elderly patients simply because of their age. As long as there are no contraindications to its use (see Chapter 8), and as long as the patient is able to comprehend the technique, PCA is a safe and effective form of pain relief. Although in general the proportion of elderly patients who can

Box 14.3

Analgesic drugs (other than opioids) and their use in the elderly

Local anesthetic drugs	Clearance may be decreased
	If repeat doses or continuous infusions are used, the total dose may need to be reduced in order to avoid possible accumulation
Non-steroidal anti-inflammatory drugs (NSAIDs) and COX-2 inhibitors	Increased risk of renal complications: the elderly are more likely to have renal impairment, cardiac failure and hypovolemia, or to be using diuretic or antihypertensive medications
	Increased risk of gastrointestinal side effects
	The incidence is increased when NSAIDs with longer half-lives are used, so these are probably best avoided in the elderly
	The incidence may be less when COX-2 inhibitors are used
	In frail elderly patients NSAIDs may cause cognitive dysfunction
Paracetamol (acetaminophen)	There is no consistent evidence regarding the effect of aging on clearance and there is probably no need to reduce doses in the elderly
Tricyclic antidepressants (TCAs)	Increased risk of side effects such as sedation, confusion, orthostatic hypotension, dry mouth, constipation and urinary retention (incidence may be highest with amitriptyline)
	Initial doses should be lower than for younger patients (i.e. 5–10 mg) and any increases should be titrated slowly
	More likely to have diseases that require TCAs to be administered with caution (e.g. prostatic hypertrophy, narrow-angle glaucoma, cardiovascular disease and impaired liver function)
Anticonvulsants	More likely to develop side effects
	Initial doses should be lower than for younger patients and any increases should be titrated slowly
	Reduction in liver function may affect elimination of drugs such as carbamazepine
	Reduction in renal function may affect the clearance of drugs such as gabapentin

(Continued)

Box 14.3—cont'd

Analgesic drugs (other than opioids) and their use in the elderly

Ketamine	Lower doses required (may be as low as 1 mg/h by infusion)
Nitrous oxide	Older patients are more likely to have a vitamin B_{12} deficiency, putting them at increased risk of a nitrous oxide-induced neuropathy

---

use PCA effectively will be smaller than in younger age groups, some patients in their 90s have been reported to do so successfully. Elderly patients should be followed closely to ensure that they understand the concept of self-administration, and to ensure that they are obtaining adequate pain relief.

In the elderly patient (over 70 years) it is suggested that the size of the PCA bolus dose be reduced. The use of a background (continuous) infusion with PCA has been shown to increase the amount of opioid delivered and increase the risk of side effects. Therefore, these are best avoided in the elderly. The opioid-tolerant patient may be an exception.

It is also wise to avoid concurrent use of drugs that depress the central nervous system, especially longer-acting sedatives such as scopolamine (hyoscine) and lorazepam. As well as increasing the risk of respiratory depression in any patient receiving opioids, they can reduce the chance of older patients remembering what they have been told about PCA and hence their ability to understand and use it appropriately. This therapy should be stopped if a patient becomes confused, as it may no longer be used correctly.

Epidural analgesia

Elderly patients are at particular risk of complications after surgery or major trauma and are therefore most likely to benefit from an analgesic technique, such as epidural analgesia, that might improve outcome (see Chapter 1). If closely supervised by an acute pain service team, with appropriate patient monitoring and staff education, even elderly patients (including those over 100) with epidural analgesia can be safely managed in general surgical wards.

As with parenteral opioids, epidural opioid requirements decrease with increasing patient age. In addition, the spread of a given volume of local anesthetic drug in the epidural space is greater in the elderly. Whether these drugs are used alone or in combination, age-based dose or infusion rate regimens are therefore recommended (see Chapter 9).

The elderly may be more at risk of some of the adverse effects of epidural analgesia (e.g. they may be less able to compensate for hypovolemia). They may also be less likely to mention side effects such as motor or sensory block or backache, which could indicate an epidural hematoma or abscess. Spinal stenosis, a common problem in the elderly, may also be a risk factor for neurological complications after epidural analgesia. Therefore, these patients need close monitoring.

As with any patient, minimization of hemodynamic change (including orthostatic hypotension), early ambulation, and early recognition of any major complication will be made easier if analgesia is titrated to provide sufficient pain relief without motor and sensory block. Appropriate placement of the epidural catheter will help to reduce the dose of drug required for effective pain relief, and therefore help to minimize side effects.

Anticoagulant drugs

It should be noted that the dose and duration of effect of anticoagulant drugs can be altered in the elderly. This may be clinically important when these drugs are used in patients receiving epidural analgesia. Low molecular weight heparins are eliminated primarily by the kidney, and so clearance is likely to be reduced in the elderly patient. Age-related reductions in warfarin requirements are also seen owing to alterations in free plasma warfarin fractions and decreased production of clotting factors. Concurrent medical problems, including cardiac and renal disease, and interactions with other drugs (both more likely in the elderly patient) can also lead to an increased sensitivity to warfarin therapy.

Key points

Evidence level

I Experimental pain thresholds to a variety of noxious stimuli are increased in elderly people, but there is also a reduction in tolerance to pain

III Reported frequency and intensity of acute pain in clinical situations may be reduced in the elderly

III Common unidimensional self-report measures of pain can be used in the elderly patient in the acute pain setting; in the clinical setting, the verbal descriptor scale may be more reliable than others

IV There is an age-related decrease in opioid requirements; significant interpatient variability persists

Clinical practice point

Measures of current pain may be more reliable than past pain, especially in patients with some cognitive impairment

Opioid-tolerant patients

In previous chapters emphasis was placed on the large interpatient variation in the amount of opioid required for effective analgesia, and the need to titrate the dose to effect for each patient. When patients have been taking opioids for a prolonged period (whether legally prescribed or illegally obtained) effective titration can be much more difficult. Many of these patients will be tolerant to and physically dependent on these drugs, and some – a much smaller proportion – will have a substance abuse disorder (SAD) involving opioids (i.e. an addiction to opioids – see next section).

The provision of effective pain relief in these patients can be difficult and challenging and may require significant deviation from standardized protocols. It is recommended that advice be obtained from pain medicine physicians and other specialists in the relevant areas. The management of a patient with a substance abuse disorder is covered in the following section.

Opioid tolerance, dependence and addiction

Tolerance

Patients on long-term opioid therapy may develop a tolerance to the drug. The term refers to the progressive decrease in analgesic effect seen for the same dose of opioid, or the need for progressively larger doses to maintain the same effect (see Box 14.4).

The mechanisms underlying the development of tolerance are still not fully understood, but they appear to overlap with those mechanisms that are thought to produce and maintain persistent pain states (see Chapter 12), and include desensitization and downregulation (i.e. a decrease in responsiveness) of μ opioid receptors and involvement of the N-methyl-D-aspartate (NMDA) receptor.

Another reason why these patients may have inadequate pain relief despite increasing doses of opioid is *opioid-induced hyperalgesia* (OIH). This means that opioids can, paradoxically, lead to increased pain sensitivity (hyperalgesia) rather than analgesia. As with persistent pain, the mechanisms underlying OIH seem to overlap with those underlying opioid tolerance. However, unlike with tolerance, increasing opioid doses will not improve analgesia. The clinical significance of this mix of tolerance and OIH is difficult to determine. With the former, higher doses would be expected to improve pain relief. If higher doses fail to provide better analgesia or if the pain appears to be getting worse, then OIH should be suspected and opioid doses reduced. It is possible that the interventions outlined below that may help to attenuate tolerance may also be effective for OIH.

Box 14.4

Definitions of tolerance, dependence and addiction

Tolerance	A decrease in sensitivity to opioids, resulting in less effect from the same dose, or the need for progressively larger doses to maintain the same effect
Physical dependence	A physiological adaptation to a drug characterized by the emergence of a withdrawal (abstinence) syndrome if the drug is abruptly stopped, reduced in dose or antagonized
Addiction	A pattern of drug use characterized by aberrant drug-taking behaviors and the compulsive use of a substance in order to experience its psychic effects, or to avoid the effects of its absence (withdrawal). There is continued use despite the risk of physical, psychological or social harm to the user
Pseudoaddiction	Drug-seeking behavior caused by a need for better pain relief

---

In the clinical setting tolerance is probably not a significant determinant of opioid requirements in most cases. Many patients on long-term opioid therapy will not require dose increases for weeks, months, or even years. If dose escalation is evident, causes other than tolerance should be considered. These include:

- Increasing pain due to disease progression (more likely in patients with cancer pain, e.g. due to disease progression)
- Pain due to postoperative complications (e.g. compartment syndrome, peritonitis)
- Onset of neuropathic pain
- Opioid-induced hyperalgesia
- Major psychological distress (e.g. anxiety, depression)
- Aberrant drug-taking behaviors (see next section).

The practical significance of opioid tolerance in acute pain management is that such patients may require much higher doses than an opioid-naive patient after a similar injury or operation. Dose regimens therefore need careful titration if effective pain relief is to be achieved. PCA may be a practical way of allowing the patient to self-titrate these doses (see below).

Tolerance also develops to opioid-related side effects, but to varying degrees and at varying rates. Tolerance to nausea and vomiting, cognitive impairment, sedation and respiratory depression occurs rapidly; tolerance to constipation and miosis develops very slowly, if at all.

Despite tolerance to the effects of opioids, side effects, including respiratory depression, can occur in opioid-tolerant patients. This is especially likely if doses are suddenly and markedly increased above usual 'baseline' levels, as might occur after surgery. In the study by Rapp and colleagues (1995), opioid-tolerant patients using PCA had a much higher incidence of sedation than those who were not opioid tolerant.

Incomplete cross-tolerance

Patients tolerant to one opioid will usually be tolerant to all other opioids. This is called cross-tolerance. However, the degree of cross-tolerance that occurs is unpredictable and appears to be incomplete. In chronic pain and palliative care settings, when a change is made from one opioid to another the new drug is often commenced at a dose that is about 50% of the calculated equianalgesic dose of the first. The same practice may be required in acute pain settings. Subsequent doses of the alternative opioid should then be titrated to effect.

If a decision is made to change opioid therapy to methadone, doses that are about 10–15% of the expected equianalgesic dose may be more appropriate. The required dose may be much lower for a number of reasons, including the long and variable half-life of methadone and its NMDA receptor antagonist and monoaminergic agonist properties.

As noted in Chapter 4, equianalgesic doses are based on single-dose studies in opioid-naive patients. The equianalgesic doses of opioids in patients on long-term therapy are unknown, and equianalgesic dose tables must be used with caution.

Opioid rotation

If pain is uncontrolled, the first step is usually to increase the dose of opioid. In some patients, especially those requiring high doses, further increases may be limited by intolerable side effects (despite aggressive treatment of the side effects) even though pain relief remains inadequate. In such patients a change to another opioid (opioid rotation), in smaller than equivalent doses, may result in better analgesia and an improved side-effect profile. The same approach can be used in patients who develop adverse effects even on relatively low doses of one opioid, but who may not experience these with another opioid.

The concept of opioid rotation is based on the belief that this change will allow clearance of the first opioid and its metabolites, and the observation that some patients tolerate one opioid much better than another. It also takes advantage of the fact that incomplete cross-tolerance is likely to exist.

If a patient requires high doses of morphine prior to surgery, high levels of morphine metabolites may already be present, particularly if the patient is taking oral morphine. Increased dose requirements in the immediate postoperative period will lead to further increases in metabolite levels, and metabolite-related side effects may then occur. In this case the use of an alternative opioid such as fentanyl to manage the acute pain episode would allow time for these metabolites to clear.

Attenuation of tolerance

There are a number of strategies that may help attenuate opioid tolerance to a certain degree and improve analgesia. Those that might be of some use in the acute pain setting include:

- The addition of non-opioids, including paracetamol and NSAIDs or coxibs
- Opioid rotation
- Use of NMDA receptor antagonists such as ketamine
- Use of regional analgesic techniques.

Ketamine (see Chapter 6) has been shown to prevent or reverse opioid tolerance in rodents, and there is some limited evidence that it may reduce opioid requirements and improve pain relief in opioid-tolerant patients.

Physical dependence

Physical dependence refers to the physiological adaptation of the CNS to opioids, characterized by the development of a withdrawal (or abstinence) syndrome if the opioid is antagonized (by opioid antagonists or agonist–antagonists), suddenly stopped, or abruptly reduced in dose. In other words, continued opioid use is required in order to suppress signs and symptoms of withdrawal (see Box 14.4). It must be emphasized that tolerance and dependence are natural biological consequences of repeated drug use and do *not* imply abuse or addiction.

The lowest dose of an opioid and the shortest duration of treatment that may lead to physical dependence are not known. Dependence should be presumed to exist if repeated doses of an opioid are given over 1–2 weeks. However, the degree of withdrawal that would be experienced if the opioid were stopped abruptly would depend on the doses that had been used.

In acute pain management the development of dependence is usually relatively unimportant. Most patients after surgery or trauma, even if opioids have been required for more than a week or two, tend to reduce their opioid intake as the pain reduces; that is, weaning from opioids occurs naturally, and in the majority of patients planned dose reductions are not required.

However, in acute pain management situations can arise when high doses of opioids are abruptly stopped or reduced. For example, a patient on long-term opioid therapy may be given epidural or intrathecal analgesia in the postoperative period. In most cases the amount of opioid delivered by these routes is relatively small and less than that required to prevent the onset of a withdrawal syndrome. Additional systemic opioids may be required.

Another example is a patient who requires high doses of opioid several days after surgery, but who is otherwise ready for discharge from hospital. In this situation, a discharge prescription may be necessary for the purpose of tapering the opioid dose, in order to prevent a withdrawal syndrome after the patient has returned home. Liaison with the patient's family practitioner may be advisable.

Withdrawal (abstinence) syndrome

Signs and symptoms of withdrawal syndrome include yawning, sweating, lacrimation, rhinorrhea, anxiety, restlessness, insomnia, dilated pupils, piloerection, chills, tachycardia, hypertension, nausea and vomiting, crampy abdominal pains, diarrhea, and muscle aches and pains. Piloerection results in the appearance of gooseflesh, so that the skin resembles that of a plucked turkey. Thus the expression 'going cold turkey' is used to describe the syndrome of abrupt withdrawal from opioids.

In patients dependent on short-acting opioids withdrawal may occur as soon as 4–6 hours after the last dose, but will occur later with the use of methadone or slow-release preparations. The prevention of withdrawal syndrome is discussed later in this chapter.

Categories of opioid-tolerant patient

Opioid-tolerant patients are often divided into three groups, those with:

- cancer pain
- chronic non-cancer pain
- a past or current addiction to opioids.

In the acute pain management setting, this grouping is not necessarily helpful. Some staff may even 'rate' patients according to group, ranging from those 'worthy of good treatment' to those 'not so worthy'. They may also have preconceived ideas about who will be a 'good' patient and easy to treat, and who is likely to be 'difficult and demanding'. These attitudes are to be strongly discouraged.

'Difficult' personalities can certainly add to the challenges of treatment, but patients may be much less 'difficult' if they perceive that staff are taking their pain reports and pain management seriously.

From a practical point of view, patients in all three groups are likely to be tolerant to and have a physical dependence on opioids. What can make effective pain management more difficult is whether these patients exhibit, or have exhibited, any aberrant drug-taking behaviors (see next section). Although these behaviors are more likely to be seen in patients with an addiction to opioids, they may be seen in some patients on long-term opioid therapy for chronic non-cancer pain, and much less commonly in patients with cancer. Particularly challenging for the treating physician is the patient with chronic pain who shows significant aberrant drug-taking behaviors, and who then has an operation or accident resulting in acute pain.

Aims of treatment

The principles of acute pain management in the opioid-tolerant patient will be similar regardless of the group to which the patient belongs. The main differences in treatment occur when the patient also exhibits some of the aberrant drug-taking behaviors described above. The main aims of treatment are summarized in Box 14.5.

Analgesia

The acute pain (the 'new' pain) needs to be brought under control as quickly and effectively as possible. A patient who has a concurrent chronic pain problem (e.g. back pain) needs to be aware that the main aim of treatment, in the first instance at least, is to manage the acute episode.

Box 14.5

Aims of treatment

- Provision of adequate analgesia
- Prevention of withdrawal
- Management of withdrawal from other drugs
- Involvement of multidisciplinary and/or other specialist teams and treatment of comorbidities (depression etc.) as needed
- Management of aberrant drug-taking behaviors

In general, multimodal analgesic regimens will be of most benefit, and the use of non-opioids and regional analgesic techniques should be maximized in these patients. However, as opioids will frequently be used in the treatment of their acute pain, most of the following discussion centers on this group of drugs. Before they are administered, the amount of opioid the patient has been taking prior to admission may need to be confirmed with the prescriber.

Well-established guidelines for acute pain management provide a useful framework for analgesic use in opioid-tolerant patients, as they do for those who are opioid-naive.

Preferred opioid

Pure opioid agonists are usually the drugs of choice at this time, as there is no ceiling to the dose that can be given in the absence of side effects. The exception is pethidine (meperidine), where doses would have to be limited because of potential problems with norpethidine (normeperidine) toxicity (see Chapter 4). Generally, pethidine is best avoided in the treatment of these, if not most, patients. Using an opioid other than the one the patient is using long term (opioid rotation) may be an advantage in some circumstances.

Doses

Opioid requirements will often be much higher than 'average' in the period immediately after surgery or major injury, but the amount needed can be difficult to judge. It may be best to start with a conservative estimate and then rapidly titrate the drug until the patient is comfortable (based on assessment criteria, including function). The dose prescribed should take into account the patient's current opioid requirement, although these estimates may be difficult to obtain when illicit drugs have been used. In the short term, and in the absence of any contraindication, the total dose may be increased until satisfactory analgesia is obtained or until side effects limit further increases. See suggestions below for ways to 'calculate' initial bolus doses for PCA.

The patient should be assured that staff will aim for good analgesia. However, safety is paramount, and the onset of sedation or other significant side effects may prevent further dose escalation. In the event that doses are increased to a level where the patient becomes sedated but still complains of pain, it should be explained that further opioid cannot be given safely. In some patients the pain may not be completely responsive to opioids, as is the case with neuropathic pain. In this case other drugs or interventional methods of pain relief may be needed.

In most cases the aim will be to discharge the patient on the dose of opioid used before admission. Such plans should be discussed with the patient at an early stage.

MONITORING FOR EFFECT AND SIDE EFFECTS In general, opioid-tolerant patients, especially those with chronic non-cancer pain or an addiction to opioids, tend to report higher pain scores. Pain scores may therefore not be a reliable guide to alterations in therapy, and high scores will not always dictate further increases in opioid dose. An objective assessment of function (e.g. ability to cough, ambulate) may be a better guide to treatment in some patients.

Ketamine

As noted earlier, the NMDA receptor is thought to be one of the factors involved in the development of tolerance, and NMDA receptor antagonist drugs such as ketamine may block or reverse that tolerance. For this reason, ketamine administered in low doses of 50–200 mg/24 hours (the lower doses used in the older patients) by IV or SC infusion may be a useful adjunct in some opioid-tolerant patients, with few, if any, side effects.

Other analgesic agents and techniques

A number of non-opioid drugs will be useful adjuvants to opioid analgesia, partly because they are analgesic in their own right and rely on mechanisms of actions unrelated to the opioid receptors. Some may even attenuate tolerance. These include clonidine and NSAIDs. Tramadol may also be of use, although its sole administration *instead* of any opioid is not recommended, as it will not prevent opioid withdrawal. In addition, the total doses required in opioid-tolerant patients may exceed recommended dose limits.

Where appropriate, regional analgesic techniques will also be of benefit. It should be remembered, however, that the doses of opioids administered by the epidural or intrathecal routes will not necessarily be enough to prevent the signs and symptoms of opioid withdrawal.

Prevention of withdrawal syndromes

If patients are unable to continue their normal chronic opioid therapy in the postoperative or post-trauma period (e.g. because they are fasting or because their 'normal' opioid is illicit), sufficient drug must be given to cover their basal requirement in order to prevent withdrawal. Basal requirements should be provided regardless of the reported pain.

If patients have required high systemic doses of opioid for the treatment of acute pain for more than a few days, they may also be at risk of withdrawal if the drug is stopped abruptly or doses reduced too rapidly. In general, reductions of about 20–25% every day or two will allow a tapering of dose without signs and symptoms of withdrawal.

More rapid tapering can be achieved if the patient is given clonidine (an α_2-adrenergic agonist, see Chapter 6). As well as its use in the treatment of hypertension and as an analgesic agent, clonidine has been used to prevent and/or treat signs and symptoms of withdrawal. Doses may start at 25–50 µg three times a day (oral or SC) and can be increased as needed. However, it must be remembered that clonidine cannot be stopped abruptly because of the risk of headache, nausea, insomnia, rebound hypertension and cardiac arrhythmias.

In patients with a substance abuse disorder, dependence on other drugs such as benzodiazepines or alcohol is common and treatment must also aim to prevent withdrawal from these drugs.

Involvement of multidisciplinary and other specialist teams

In many of these patients, management of behavioral, psychological, medical and other factors may be needed in addition to analgesia. Assistance from other specialist teams, including chronic pain, palliative care, drug and alcohol, and psychiatric services, may be advisable.

Opioid-tolerant patients may have significant emotional and psychiatric comorbidities that require treatment. Patients with cancer pain, for example, may suffer from depression. This may be exacerbated if the acute pain for which they are now being treated serves to remind them of their limited life expectancy (e.g. if pain signifies disease progression, or if the operation has been for palliation only). Common comorbidities in patients who abuse drugs or alcohol are depression, anxiety, and borderline personality disorders. These too can be exacerbated during the acute pain episode.

Specific analgesic techniques

Patient-controlled analgesia

If patients are unable to continue their normal chronic opioid medication (e.g. because they are fasting), a continuous (background) infusion can be used to cover this basal requirement, allowing for incomplete cross-tolerance where appropriate.

Larger-than-average bolus doses will often be needed, although it can be difficult to know the optimal starting dose. One method is to base the size of the bolus dose (as well as any background infusion) on the patient's normal (preadmission) opioid requirement. Examples of this are given below. These examples are based on patients in whom good pain relief was obtained when 'standard' PCA protocols were adapted to suit them. The dose regimens are suggestions only and may not be suitable for all patients or in all situations. The use of higher bolus doses is best limited to situations where the patient is being managed by specialist pain services, when there is 24-hour (appropriate) medical cover, when nursing and medical staff have had appropriate education and experience, and when adequate monitoring is available.

Example 1

Following laparotomy, a patient is offered morphine PCA. For the last 8 months he has been taking 300 mg of a controlled-release oral morphine preparation (in divided doses) daily. He is not permitted any oral intake after the operation.

basal opioid requirement	= 300 mg/day oral morphine
using a 3:1 conversion	= 100 mg/day IV morphine
	= 4 mg/h approximately
therefore, appropriate background infusion	= 4 mg/h
bolus dose	= 4 mg

Example 2

A patient will receive morphine PCA after surgery for multiple injuries. For the last 6 months he has been taking 800 mg of a controlled-release oral morphine preparation (in divided doses) daily. He is not permitted any oral intake after the operation.

basal opioid requirement	= 800 mg/day oral morphine
	= 260 mg/day IV morphine
approximately	= 10 mg/h

It is thought appropriate to use another opioid in the immediate postoperative period (see previous comments about incomplete cross-tolerance and morphine metabolites). The decision is made to use fentanyl.

The equianalgesic dose of 10 mg morphine would normally be considered to be about 150–200 μg fentanyl (see Chapter 4). As cross-tolerance is likely to be incomplete, doses of 50% of the equianalgesic dose could be used initially, therefore:

| background infusion | = 100 μg/h approximately |
| bolus dose | = 100 μg |

Doses and infusion rates may require adjustment (up or down) according to pain relief or side effects. As a general rule it may be best to keep the rate of infusion (in mg/h) the same as or less than the size of the bolus dose (in mg), so that PCA remains predominantly 'patient controlled'.

If a patient is taking methadone on a regular basis, it is more difficult to calculate an appropriate initial PCA bolus dose because the very variable half-life of methadone and its long duration of action make any estimate of true 'equianalgesic' dose almost impossible. In practice it seems reasonable to use a 1:1 conversion in the initial stage of treatment and then thereafter to adjust PCA regimens to suit.

If parenteral methadone is available, it can be run as an infusion at a rate equivalent to about 75% of the oral dose. If parenteral methadone is not available, an alternative opioid will need to be used as a background infusion.

Example 3

For the last 3 years a patient he has been taking 100 mg of methadone daily. He is not permitted any oral intake after the operation. The decision is made to use morphine.

basal opioid requirement	= 100 mg/day oral morphine
using a 1:1 conversion	= 100 mg/day IV morphine
bolus dose	= 4 mg morphine
If parenteral methadone is available:	= 3 mg/h by (separate) infusion *or*
If parenteral methadone not available:	= 4 mg/h morphine as a PCA background infusion

---

Note: If a patient's usual opioid requirements are much greater than those in the above examples, it may be wise to be more conservative and start at lower than calculated doses and background infusion rates.

Once the patient is tolerating unlimited oral fluids, usual opioid regimens can be restarted to replace the background infusion. In addition, short-term use of immediate-release opioids, such as morphine, oxycodone or hydromorphone, may be needed. High PCA dose requirements may mean that there is a delay before the patient can be managed with their usual opioids alone.

Addiction to opioids (see next section) was initially believed to be a contraindication to the use of PCA. However, it is now recognized as a potentially useful method of providing pain relief in these patients. This is partly because of the possibility of large opioid requirements and partly because it helps avoid confrontations between staff and patients.

The central assumptions behind the use of PCA are that a patient will self-administer opioid when uncomfortable, and when comfort is achieved will make no further demands. The advantages of PCA are lost if the patient uses the pump simply to self-administer as much opioid as the settings allow. They should be reminded to use PCA for pain control only and not for other reasons.

Regional analgesia

A variety of regional analgesic techniques, including epidural and intrathecal analgesia, and continuous brachial plexus or lumbar plexus blocks, may be used to provide safe and effective pain relief in opioid-dependent patients.

Replacement of basal opioid requirements will be needed in order to prevent signs and symptoms of opioid withdrawal. If an opioid is added to the epidural infusion, the amount delivered may or may not be adequate for this purpose and this should be calculated for every patient. The amount of opioid administered for intrathecal analgesia (commonly 0.1–0.2 mg morphine) will usually be inadequate.

Key points

Evidence level

III Opioid-tolerant patients report higher pain scores and have a lower incidence of opioid-induced nausea and vomiting

IV Ketamine may reduce opioid requirements in opioid-tolerant patients

Clinical practice points

Usual preadmission opioid regimens should be maintained where possible, or appropriate substitutions made

Opioid-tolerant patients are at risk of opioid withdrawal if non-opioid analgesic regimens or tramadol alone are used

PCA settings may need to include a background infusion to replace the usual opioid dose and a higher bolus dose

Neuraxial opioids can be used effectively in opioid-tolerant patients, although higher doses may be required and these may be inadequate to prevent withdrawal

Reproduced with permission from Acute Pain Management: Scientific Evidence ANZCA and FPM (2005).

Patients with a substance abuse disorder

Patients who have a substance abuse disorder (SAD) involving opioids (i.e. are addicted to opioids – see definition, Box 14.4) will usually be tolerant to their effects and physically dependent on the drugs, although this need not be the case. Management may be complicated by associated psychological and behavioral factors, by the presence of other drugs of abuse or medications that assist with drug withdrawal and/or rehabilitation, and by possible complications related to drug abuse, including infectious diseases. In some patients concerns may arise because of the difficulty of balancing anxieties about the undertreatment of pain against safety and possible diversion of the drug.

It is their aberrant drug-taking behavioral patterns and loss of personal control that distinguish patients with a SAD from other patients on long-term opioid therapy. A wide variety of aberrant drug-taking behaviors have been described, some of which are said to be less common but more suggestive of addiction (Box 14.6); others are more common but less suggestive of addiction (Box 14.7). The latter are more likely to reflect undertreated distress of some kind (e.g. pain or psychological distress). Patients who are anxious, depressed, or have borderline personality disorders may exhibit some aberrant drug-taking behaviors.

Patients with a SAD have both a physical and a psychological need for the drug. Compulsive use of that drug occurs despite the risk of physical, psychological or social harm. Commonly, such patients are willing to acquire the drug by deception or by illegal means. Close liaison with drug and alcohol services and other treating clinicians is recommended.

If a patient with a SAD involving opioids is not already in an addiction treatment program, the immediate postoperative or post-injury period is probably not the time to discuss the various options. It is better to gain the confidence of the patient by providing good analgesia and to leave any discussion about treatment of addiction until later.

Pseudoaddiction

Occasionally, staff may report that a patient is 'becoming addicted' to opioids when they appear to be demanding pain-relieving drugs and

---

Box 14.6

Drug-taking behaviors that may be suggestive of addiction

- Polysubstance use/abuse (e.g. alcohol, sedatives)
- Seeking drugs from other medical sources (e.g. forging or altering prescriptions, 'doctor shopping', 'lost' prescriptions)
- Seeking drugs from non-medical sources (e.g. stealing, borrowing, illegal sources of medical or illicit drugs)
- Multiple unsanctioned dose escalations or other non-compliance with treatment
- Deteriorating ability to function at work or socially
- Diversion of drugs (e.g. selling the drugs)
- Injection of oral preparations of a drug (e.g. methadone syrup)

Data from Passik and Portenoy (1998).

Box 14.7

Drug-taking behaviors that are less suggestive of addiction

- One or two unsanctioned dose escalations or other non-compliance with treatment
- Use of the drug to treat other symptoms
- Complaints (sometimes aggressive) about the need for higher doses
- Attempts to negotiate treatment
- Requesting or demanding specific drugs
- Hoarding drugs

Data from Passik and Portenoy (1998).

exhibiting aberrant drug-taking behaviors similar to those seen in patients with an addiction. However, patients may seek or demand more analgesia if pain relief is inadequate. Undertreatment of acute pain may lead to iatrogenic drug-seeking behaviors that are really pain-avoidance behaviors. Weisman and Haddox (1989) termed this *pseudoaddiction*.

Use of opioids in patients with a past SAD

If a patient has had a past SAD involving opioids there may be concern that the use of opioids for analgesia will lead to the reinstatement of a craving for drugs. Whereas local anesthetic blocks and NSAIDs may suffice in some patients, the primary concern must still be good pain relief. If opioids are indicated they should be used in effective doses because ineffective analgesia may lead to anxiety and drug-seeking behaviors and demands, as well as pain.

Those who abuse opioids generally seek a change in mental status and euphoria. The more rapidly this can be achieved, the more desirable it becomes. In patients who exhibit aberrant drug-taking behaviors, drug and dose regimens that minimize large and rapid swings in blood levels may be preferred. For example, PCA may be preferable to larger IV bolus doses or IM injections of an opioid.

Management of withdrawal from other drugs

It is not uncommon for patients who have an addiction to opioids to be addicted to other drugs as well (e.g. alcohol, barbiturates or benzodiazepines). Monitoring of signs and symptoms that indicate withdrawal from these drugs is suggested, and prevention or treatment regimens should be instituted as necessary.

Signs and symptoms of withdrawal from alcohol include anxiety, agitation, restlessness, sleep disturbances, nausea and vomiting, hallucinations, confusion, disorientation and seizures. These usually occur 12–48 hours after the last intake of alcohol. Signs and symptoms of withdrawal from benzodiazepines are similar, but onset may be delayed for 1–5 days.

If patients are withdrawing from drugs that put them at risk of seizures, other drugs that are known to lower the seizure threshold (e.g. tricyclic antidepressants, tramadol) should be used with care.

Withdrawal from stimulant drugs such as amfetamine (amphetamine) can lead to marked sedation and consequent difficulties in safely obtaining adequate analgesia with opioids.

Management of aberrant drug-taking behaviors

Individualized treatment plans that help with effective and safe yet compassionate treatment can benefit patients who may exhibit significant aberrant drug-taking behaviors (e.g. those currently abusing drugs or alcohol, those who have done so in the past, and those in drug treatment programs).

These treatment plans, which should be firmly applied, may include realistic goals for analgesia (complete pain relief is usually not realistic), expected duration of treatment, plans for dose reductions and choice of drugs available. The dangers associated with tampering with equipment, or the use of illicit drugs in addition to prescribed medications, should also be explained. All medical and nursing staff involved in treating the patient should agree with and adhere to the plans, which should also be discussed with the patient.

Drugs used in the treatment of substance abuse disorders

Methadone

Methadone is a long-acting pure opioid agonist often used in the management of patients with an opioid SAD. In the acute pain setting, if the patient cannot take their usual oral methadone, substitution with parenteral methadone or another pure opioid agonist will be needed.

Naltrexone

Naltrexone (see Chapter 4) is used in the treatment of an opioid or alcohol SAD.

It may be difficult to achieve adequate pain relief with opioid drugs, even in high doses, until the effects of naltrexone have weakened. Therefore, where possible, naltrexone should be ceased at least 24 hours prior to surgery. There is some evidence that patients may be more sensitive to opioids following cessation of naltrexone, therefore they should be monitored closely if other opioid analgesia is given during this time.

Alternative analgesic drugs (e.g. ketamine, NSAIDs) and techniques (e.g. local anesthetic blocks) should be used where indicated.

Buprenorphine

Buprenorphine is a partial opioid agonist (see Chapter 4) that is also increasingly being used in the treatment of an opioid SAD. As yet, there is no good evidence on which to base the management of acute pain in these patients.

If the buprenorphine were to be stopped, a change to an alternative opioid such as methadone would be needed to prevent withdrawal. This could take days or weeks. In practice, there appears to be little problem if the buprenorphine is continued and acute pain managed with the combination of a pure agonist opioid (e.g. fentanyl) in doses based on the dose of buprenorphine, as well as other multimodal analgesic regimens.

Key points

Clinical practice points

Naltrexone should be stopped at least 24 hours before elective surgery

Patients who have completed naltrexone therapy should be regarded as opioid naive; in the immediate post-treatment phase they may be opioid sensitive

Maintenance methadone regimens should be continued where possible

Buprenorphine maintenance may be continued; if buprenorphine is ceased prior to surgery conversion to an alternative opioid is required

Reproduced with permission from Acute Pain Management: Scientific Evidence ANZCA and FPM (2005).

Patients with obstructive sleep apnea

The prevalence of obstructive sleep apnea (OSA) in the adult population is surprisingly high: approximately one in five adults has at least mild OSA, and one in 15 has moderate to severe OSA. Importantly in the acute pain setting, around three-quarters of those who could benefit from treatment remain undiagnosed.

There is little good evidence to guide the 'best choice' of acute pain management regimen in patients with OSA. Non-opioid analgesics and regional analgesic techniques are usually recommended, either as the sole means of pain relief or in addition to opioids, because of concerns that the patient with OSA is at increased risk of opioid-induced respiratory depression and hypoxia if given opioid or sedative drugs.

However, many patients who have undiagnosed OSA will be given opioids for the management of their acute pain. It is therefore essential that any opioid administered to any patient is titrated safely. This requires the use of appropriate doses, the avoidance of a background infusion with PCA (at least in the initial stages of therapy, or unless the patient is opioid tolerant), close monitoring of the patient's level of sedation, and a reduction in opioid dose should the patient become excessively sedated (sedation score = 2 or 3), regardless of their level of pain.

Supplemental oxygen given to patients with OSA (not in a perioperative setting) has been shown to be as effective as CPAP (continuous positive airway pressure) in reducing the risk of significant hypoxemia. The routine use of supplemental oxygen would therefore seem appropriate in all patients with OSA (or suspected of having OSA) and receiving opioids for the treatment of their pain.

Opioid analgesia and patients with OSA

A number of studies investigating hypoxia in postoperative patients without OSA have shown that opioid administration leads to recurrent episodes of upper airway obstruction when the patient is asleep. This would suggest that concerns about an increased risk of upper airway obstruction after opioid administration in patients with OSA are reasonable.

Although the effects of opioids on upper airway obstruction have not yet been formally studied in patients with OSA, there have been a number of case reports of life-threatening or fatal respiratory depression following PCA, epidural and intramuscular opioid administration in these patients.

However, when these reports are studied in detail, it is obvious that one of the main problems was the lack of appropriate monitoring to detect impending respiratory depression. Inappropriate dose regimens also appeared to contribute in some patients (e.g. use of a background infusion with PCA).

It is known that increasing sedation is the best early clinical indicator of respiratory depression (see Chapter 3), and yet it would seem, in most if not all of the reports, that inappropriate reliance was placed on monitoring the patient's respiratory rate. In many of the reports, marked sedation and hypercarbia were noted in the presence of a normal respiratory rate. Had sedation levels been monitored, and had appropriate opioid dose reductions been made when excessive sedation was first noticed, it may be that the problems could have been detected at an earlier stage and severe respiratory depression averted.

Key points

Evidence level

III Patients with OSA may be at higher risk of complications after surgery and from opioid analgesia

Clinical practice point

Management strategies that may increase the efficacy and safety of pain relief in patients with OSA include the provision of appropriate multimodal opioid-sparing analgesia, CPAP, monitoring and supervision (in a high-dependency area if necessary), and supplemental oxygen

Reproduced with permission from Acute Pain Management: Scientific Evidence ANZCA and FPM (2005).

Pregnant or lactating patients

Analgesic use during pregnancy

The pregnant woman may require treatment for acute pain for many reasons other than during labor and delivery. The major concern in these patients is that the analgesics given to them will almost invariably cross the placenta to some degree. Where possible, non-pharmacological therapies should be used. However, if this is not possible, drugs that pose the least risk to the fetus should be prescribed.

In many countries, drugs that might be prescribed during pregnancy have been categorized according to risk. These published recommendations should be consulted before any analgesic drug is used in the pregnant patient. Although the details in each category may vary from country to country, certain generalizations can be made:

- Paracetamol (acetaminophen) is the analgesic of choice.
- Opioids can be used if the benefits are considered to outweigh the risks; these are drugs that may cause harmful effects (which may be reversible) to the human fetus or neonate because of their pharmacological actions (including withdrawal from opioids after delivery) without causing fetal malformations.
- NSAIDS given during pregnancy are associated with an increased risk of miscarriage; they should be used with caution in the last trimester as they can cause fetal cardiac and renal problems and impair the production of amniotic fluid; they should be avoided after the 32nd week.
- Withdrawal from antidepressant agents (tricyclic and SSRIs) has been reported in the neonates of mothers taking these medications.

- The anticonvulsants carbamazepine, phenytoin and sodium valproate should be avoided in pregnancy as they can cause fetal malformations.
- Of the antiemetics, metoclopramide is the drug of choice.

Analgesic use during lactation

Many of the analgesic drugs that might be prescribed during lactation will transfer in part to human milk and then to the breastfed infant. The amount transferred will be greater for those drugs that are highly lipid soluble, have a low molecular weight and are minimally protein bound.

Before analgesic drugs are prescribed for the lactating patient, it is best to consult specialist information services. However, in general, most opioids (pethidine is best avoided), paracetamol, NSAIDs (ibuprofen may be preferred, aspirin should be avoided), local anesthetics, most antidepressants and many anticonvulsants may be used safely.

As a general precaution, however, it may be best to avoid breastfeeding at times of peak maternal blood concentrations of any drug, and the

Key points

Evidence level

III Use of non-steroidal anti-inflammatory drugs during pregnancy is associated with increased risk of miscarriage

III Use of opioids in pregnancy does not cause fetal malformations, but may result in neonatal abstinence syndrome

Clinical practice points

For pain management in pregnancy non-pharmacological treatment options should be considered where possible before analgesic medications are used

Use of medications for pain in pregnancy should be guided by published recommendations; ongoing analgesic use requires close liaison between the obstetrician and the medical practitioner managing the pain

NSAIDs should be used with caution in the last trimester of pregnancy and should be avoided after the 32nd week

Prescribing medications during lactation requires consideration of possible transfer into breast milk, uptake by the baby, and potential adverse effects for the baby; it should follow available prescribing guidelines

Local anesthetics, paracetamol and several NSAIDs, in particular ibuprofen, are considered to be safe in the lactating patient

Morphine, fentanyl and oxycodone are also considered safe in the lactating patient and should be preferred to pethidine

Reproduced with permission from Acute Pain Management: Scientific Evidence ANZCA and FPM (2005).

infant should be monitored for any adverse effects of the agents that might be transferred in breast milk.

Patients with renal or hepatic impairment

In patients with renal or hepatic impairment, altered clearance of some analgesic agents or accumulation of their active metabolites may occur. This may influence the choice of drug or the dose used. Other drugs may exacerbate existing impairment.

Although good evidence is sometimes lacking regarding some of the drugs used for pain relief in these patients, certain generalizations can be made. These are summarized in Box 14.8.

Box 14.8

Analgesic drugs and their use in patients with renal or hepatic impairment

Patients with renal impairment

Opioids	*No dose adjustment required*:
	fentanyl (no active metabolites)
	oxycodone (weakly active metabolite with minimal clinical effect)
	buprenorphine (weakly active metabolites)
	Dose adjustment suggested:
	tramadol
	methadone (if impairment severe)
	Alternative agent may be preferred:
	morphine, hydromorphone, codeine
	Avoid:
	pethidine, dextropropoxyphene
Local anesthetic drugs	No significant difference in plasma concentrations of most local anesthetics; risk of toxicity could be affected by changes in acid–base status
Non-steroidal anti-inflammatory drugs(NSAIDs) and COX-2 inhibitors	*Mild renal impairment* use with caution *Severe renal impairment* avoid
Paracetamol (acetaminophen)	Safe to use

(Continued)

Box 14.8—cont'd

Tricyclic antidepressants (TCAs)	Metabolite accumulation may occur and increase the risk of side effects
Anticonvulsants	*Gabapentin* Dose adjustment suggested based on creatinine clearance
Ketamine	Limited data but probably no dose adjustment needed, especially with low-dose regimens

Patients with hepatic impairment

Opioids	*No dose adjustment required*: fentanyl, morphine *Dose adjustment may be needed:* tramadol, dextropropoxyphene *Alternative agent suggested:* methdone (if impairment severe) *Avoid:* pethidine
Local anesthetic drugs	Dose adjustment may be required with prolonged use
Non-steroidal anti-inflammatory drugs (NSAIDs) and COX-2 inhibitors	Reduced doses suggested
Paracetamol (acetaminophen)	Use with caution or in reduced doses in patients with active liver disease, alcohol-related liver and disease glucose-6-phosphate dehydrogenase deficiency
Tricyclic antidepressants (TCAs)	Limited informtion
Anticonvulsants	*Carbamazepine, valproate* Dose adjustments may be required. Not recommended in patients with severe hepatic impairment
Ketamine	Limited information

Adapted from Acute Pain Management: Scientific Evidence ANZCA and FPM (2005).

References and further reading

Abbey J, Piller N, De Bellis A et al. (2004) The Abbey pain scale: a 1-minute numerical indicator for people with end-stage dementia. International Journal of Palliative Nursing 10: 6–13.

Aubrun F. (2005) Management of postoperative analgesia in elderly patients. Regional Anesthesia and Pain Medicine 30: 363–79.

Australian and New Zealand College of Anaesthetists, Faculty of Pain Medicine (ANZCA, FPM). Acute Pain Management: Scientific Evidence, 2nd edn. 2005. Melbourne: Australian and New Zealand College of Anaesthetists, Also available online at: *http://www.anzca.edu.au/ publications/acutepain.htm* and *http://www7.health.gov.au/ nhmrc/publications/synopses/cp104syn.htm*

Bar-Oz B, Bulkowstein M, Benyamini L et al. (2003) Use of antibiotic and analgesic drugs during lactation. Drug Safety 26: 925–35.

Carroll IR, Angst MS, Clark JD. (2004) Management of perioperative pain in patients chronically consuming opioids. Regional Anesthesia and Pain Medicine 29: 576–91.

Catley DM, Thornton C, Jordan C et al. (1985) Pronounced, episodic oxygen desaturation in the postoperative period: its association with ventilatory pattern and analgesic regimen. Anesthesiology 63: 20–8.

Davies JJ, Swenson JD, Hall RH et al. (2005) Preoperative 'fentanyl challenge' as a tool to estimate postoperative opioid dosing in chronic opioid-consuming patients. Anesthesia and Analgesia 101: 389–95.

Fong HK, Sands LP, Leung JM. (2006) The role of postoperative analgesia in delirium and cognitive decline in elderly patients: a systematic review. Anesthesia and Analgesia 102: 1255–66.

Gagliese L, Weizblit N, Ellis W et al. (2005) The measurement of postoperative pain: a comparison of intensity scales in younger and older surgical patients. Pain 117: 412–20.

Gibson SJ, Farrell M. (2004) A review of age differences in the neurophysiology of nociception and the perceptual experience of pain. Clinical Journal of Pain 20: 227–39.

Gibson SJ. (2003) Pain and aging: the pain experience over the adult life span. In: Dostrovsky JO, Carr DB, Koltzenburg M, eds. Proceedings of the 10th World Congress on Pain. Seattle: IASP Press.

Herr K, Bjoro K, Decker S. (2006) Tools for assessment of pain in nonverbal adults with dementia. A state of the art review. Journal of Pain and Symptom Management 31: 170–92.

Jage J, Bey T. (2000) Postoperative analgesia in patients with substance use disorders: Part I. Acute Pain 3: 29–44.

Jage J, Bey T. (2000) Postoperative analgesia in patients with substance use disorders: Part II. Acute Pain 3: 20–8.

Kissin I, Bright CA, Bradley EL Jr. (2000) The effect of ketamine on opioid-induced acute tolerance: can it explain reduction of opioid consumption with ketamine–opioid analgesic combinations? Anesthesia and Analgesia 91: 1483–8.

Kopf A, Banzhaf A, Stein C. (2005) Perioperative management of the chronic pain patient. Best Practice and Research in Clinical Anaesthesiology 19: 59–76.

Loadsman JA, Hillman DR. (2001) Anaesthesia and sleep apnoea. British Journal of Anaesthesia 86: 254–66.

Macintyre PE, Jarvis DA. (1996) Age is the best predictor of postoperative morphine requirement. Pain 64: 357–64.

Macintyre PE, Ludbrook GL, Upton R. (2003) Acute pain in the elderly. In: Rowbotham D, Macintyre P, eds. Clinical pain management: acute volume. London: Arnold.

Macintyre PE. (2001) Safety and efficacy of patient-controlled analgesia. British Journal of Anaesthesia 87: 36–46.

Macintyre PE. (2005) Intravenous patient-controlled analgesia: one size does not fit all. Anesthesiology Clinics of North America. 23: 109–23.

Mao J. (2002) Opioid-induced abnormal pain sensitivity: implications in opioid therapy. Pain 100: 213–17.

Mehta V, Langford RM. (2006) Acute pain management in opioid dependent patients. Anaesthesia 61: 269–76.

Mitra S, Sinatra RS. (2004) Perioperative management of acute pain in the opioid-dependent patient. Anesthesiology 101: 212–27.

Murphy EJ. (2005) Acute pain management pharmacology for the patient with concurrent renal or hepatic disease. Anaesthesia and Intensive Care 33: 311–22.

Olorunto WA, Galandiuk S. (2006) Managing the spectrum of surgical pain: acute management of the chronic pain patient. Journal of the American College of Surgeons 202: 169–75.

Parikh SS, Chung FC. (1995) Postoperative delirium in the elderly. Anesthesia and Analgesia 80: 1223–31.

Passik SD, Portenoy RK. (1998) Substance abuse issues. In: Ashburn MA, Rice LJ, eds. The management of pain. Philadelphia: Churchill Livingstone.

Porter J, Jick H. (1980) Addiction rare in patients treated with narcotics. New England Journal of Medicine 302: 123.

Rapp SE, Ready LB, Nessly ML. (1995) Acute pain management in patients with prior opioid consumption: a case-controlled retrospective review. Pain 61: 195–201.

Rathmell JP, Viscomi CM, Ashburn MA. (1997) Management of nonobstetric pain during pregnancy and lactation. Anesthesia and Analgesia 85: 1074–87.

Ready LB, Chadwick HS, Ross B. (1987) Age predicts effective epidural morphine dose after abdominal hysterectomy. Anesthesia and Analgesia 66: 1215–18.

Savage SR. (2002) Assessment for addiction in pain-treatment settings. Clinical Journal of Pain 18. S28–38.

Schug SA, Morgan J. (2004) Treatment of cancer pain: special considerations in patients with renal disease. American Journal of Cancer 3: 247–56.

Spigset O, Hagg S. (2000) Analgesics and breast-feeding: safety considerations. Paediatric Drugs 2: 223–38.

Tsui BC, Wagner A, Finucane B. (2004) Regional anaesthesia in the elderly: a clinical guide. Drugs Aging 21: 895–910.

Vaurio LE, Sands LP, Wang Y et al. (2006) Postoperative delirium: the importance of pain and pain management. Anesthesia and Analgesia 102: 1267–73.

Warden V, Hurley AC, Volicer L. (2003) Development and psychometric evaluation of the Pain Assessment in Advanced Dementia (PAINAD) scale. Journal of the American Medical Directors Association 4: 9–15.

Weisman DE, Haddox JD. (1989) Opioid pseudoaddiction: an iatrogenic syndrome. Pain 36: 363–6.

Wunsch MJ, Stanard V, Schnoll SH. (2003) Treatment of pain in pregnancy. Clinical Journal of Pain 19: 148–55.

Young T, Skatrud J, Peppard PE. (2004) Risk factors for obstructive sleep apnea in adults. Journal of the American Medical Association 291: 2013–16.

Self-assessment questions

As noted in Chapter 2, nursing education and accreditation programs are important if acute pain is to be managed safely and effectively. In particular, such programs are recommended if more advanced techniques such as patient-controlled and epidural analgesia are to be made available on general hospital wards. The questions below are examples of ones that might be used as part of an accreditation assessment.

Select the ONE BEST ANSWER from the four options listed for each question.

1. Potential adverse effects of pain after surgery include:

   a. decreased myocardial oxygen consumption
   b. hypoxemia
   c. hypotension
   d. increased intestinal motility

2. Simple methods of pain relief can be more effective if there is:

   a. appropriate staff and patient education
   b. provision of appropriate guidelines and policies
   c. regular patient assessment and individualization of treatment
   d. all of the above

3. Unreliable measures of pain include:

   a. observation of patient behavior
   b. the verbal numerical rating scale
   c. the verbal descriptor scale
   d. the visual analog scale

4. The most reliable clinical indicator of opioid-induced respiratory depression is:

   a. a decrease in respiratory rate
   b. increasing sedation
   c. increasing confusion
   d. hypoxemia

5. Causes of low oxygen saturation levels in the postoperative period include all of the following EXCEPT:

   a. rebound REM sleep
   b. postoperative changes in lung function
   c. anemia
   d. opioid-related obstructive apnea

6. A patient wakes easily when you go to give him his medications. He stays awake while you are talking to him. His sedation score is:

   a. 0
   b. 1
   c. 2
   d. 3

7. A patient is wide awake and has been watching television all afternoon. His sedation score is:

   a. 0
   b. 1
   c. 2
   d. 3

8. A patient wakes easily when you go to give him his medications but appears drowsy and keeps falling asleep while you are talking to him. His sedation score is:

   a. 0
   b. 1
   c. 2
   d. 3

9. Effects of opioid receptor activation include:

   a. physical dependence, mediated via the μ receptor
   b. pruritus, mediated via the κ receptor
   c. respiratory depression, mediated via the δ receptor
   d. nausea and vomiting, mediated via the κ receptor

10. Effective antiemetic drugs in the postoperative setting include all of the following EXCEPT:

    a. droperidol
    b. dexamethasone
    c. ondansetron
    d. metoclopramide

11. The best predictor of the amount of morphine a patient is likely to need after major surgery is:

    a. gender
    b. age
    c. weight
    d. estimated lean body weight

12. If an injection of morphine is given IV, the average time for the full effect of the morphine to be seen is:

    a. 30 seconds
    b. 1 minute
    c. 5 minutes
    d. 15 minutes

13. If an injection of fentanyl is given IV, the average time for the full effect of the fentanyl to be seen is:

    a. 30 seconds
    b. 1 minute
    c. 5 minutes
    d. 15 minutes

14. Morphine 6-glucuronide (M6G) is a metabolite of morphine. M6G:

    a. may lead to hyperalgesia and allodynia
    b. does not accumulate in renal failure
    c. has analgesic activity
    d. has a shorter half-life than morphine

15. Codeine is a naturally occurring alkaloid of opium. Codeine:

    a. will not result in effective analgesia in over 50% of white patients
    b. has a high affinity for the opioid receptor
    c. is useful for the treatment of severe pain
    d. is metabolized in the liver, where about 2–10% is converted to morphine

16. Norpethidine (normeperidine) is a metabolite of pethidine. Early signs and symptoms of norpethidine toxicity:

    a. include sedation
    b. include anxiety
    c. are reversible using naloxone
    d. result from activation of opioid receptors

17. The following statements about tramadol are all true EXCEPT:
    a. the analgesic effect of tramadol is mediated only via its action on opioid receptors
    b. it causes less sedation than other opioids
    c. has an active metabolite (M1) that is dependent on the kidney for excretion
    d. it is an effective treatment in neuropathic pain

18. The following statements about buprenorphine are all true EXCEPT:
    a. it is a partial agonist drug
    b. in case of an overdose, higher than usual doses of naloxone may be required
    c. it is effective if given orally and swallowed
    d. it is available as a transdermal preparation for the management of chronic and cancer pain

19. A patient is taking 300 mg/day of a slow-release oral morphine preparation. On average, this would be equivalent to:
    a. 300 mg IV morphine
    b. 150 mg IV morphine
    c. 100 mg IV morphine
    d. 50 mg IV morphine

20. A patient is taking 200 mg/day of a slow-release oxycodone preparation. On average, this would be equivalent to:
    a. 200 mg IV morphine
    b. 150 mg IV morphine
    c. 100 mg IV morphine
    d. 50 mg IV morphine

21. A patient is taking 16 mg/day of SL buprenorphine, as part of his addiction treatment program. On average, this would be equivalent to:
    a. 200 mg IV morphine
    b. 150 mg IV morphine
    c. 100 mg IV morphine
    d. 50 mg IV morphine

22. The following statements about bupivacaine are true EXCEPT:
    a. it has a greater potential for cardiotoxicity than ropivacaine
    b. when used in low doses for regional analgesia there are no consistent differences between bupivacaine and ropivacaine in terms of quality of analgesia or motor block
    c. the addition of epinephrine (adrenaline) has little effect on the duration of action of bupivacaine given epidurally
    d. it is easier to treat cardiotoxicity following bupivacaine than following ropivacaine

23. Paracetamol (acetaminophen):

   a. should be used with caution in patients with renal impairment
   b. must not be given in doses of greater than 4 g/day
   c. has analgesic, antipyretic and anti-inflammatory activity
   d. is no more effective when given by the rectal route rather than the oral route

24. Non-steroidal anti-inflammatory drugs (NSAIDs):

   a. should be used with caution in patients with renal impairment
   b. should not be given concurrently with paracetamol
   c. result in fewer side effects when given by the rectal route rather than the oral route
   d. are more effective when given by the rectal route rather than the oral route

25. Risk factors for the development of renal failure in association with the use of NSAIDs include all of the following EXCEPT:

   a. hypotension
   b. low urine output
   c. concurrent administration of amoxicillin
   d. concurrent use of gentamicin

26. Risk factors for the development of gastric erosions following the use of NSAIDs include:

   a. concurrent use of misoprostol
   b. history of peptic ulcer disease
   c. the use of the oral rather the rectal or intravenous routes for administration of the drugs
   d. all of the above

27. Selective COX-2 inhibitors:

   a. are more effective analgesics than non-selective NSAIDs
   b. have the same risk of renal failure as non-selective NSAIDs
   c. have the same risk of bleeding as non-selective NSAIDs
   d. should not be used in patients with aspirin-exacerbated respiratory disease

28. Nitrous oxide is sometimes used as analgesia for short painful procedures. Contraindications to the use of nitrous oxide include all of the following EXCEPT:

   a. concurrent use of opioids
   b. vitamin B_{12} deficiency
   c. pneumothorax
   d. bowel obstruction

29. Ketamine:

  a. acts on NMDA receptors
  b. is ineffective in the treatment of neuropathic pain
  c. increases tolerance to opioids
  d. has a high incidence of central nervous system side effects when used in low doses (e.g. 100 mg/day)

30. The following are true about amitriptyline EXCEPT:

  a. it should be used with caution in patients with cardiac conduction abnormalities
  b. it is ineffective in the treatment of neuropathic pain
  c. it commonly causes sedation
  d. it should be started in low doses

31. Controlled-release tablets of oral morphine:

  a. take 3 hours or more to reach peak blood levels after administration
  b. are ordered '4-hourly PRN'
  c. are suitable for the rapid titration of pain relief
  d. are more potent than morphine syrup (i.e. a smaller dose is needed to give the same analgesic effect)

32. A patient is prescribed 50 mg bd slow-release oral morphine for cancer pain. An appropriate breakthrough dose of immediate-release morphine syrup would be:

  a. 1 mg
  b. 5 mg
  c. 10 mg
  d. 50 mg

33. When morphine is given by intermittent SC injection:

  a. absorption into the bloodstream will be slower than following an IM injection
  b. higher doses of morphine will be needed than if given by IM injection
  c. it should be given in the smallest volume possible
  d. repeat injections must not be given for another 4 hours

34. A 23-year-old patient is prescribed '7.5–15 mg SC morphine 1–2-hourly PRN' for pain relief after a laparotomy for a ruptured spleen the day before. He is wide awake and watching television. His last injection of morphine was 12.5 mg 90 minutes ago. He says his pain score is 9 and that he would like another injection of morphine. You would:

  a. suggest he wait another 30 minutes
  b. give 15 mg morphine
  c. give 10.0 mg morphine
  d. give 2.5 mg morphine

35. A patient who is wide awake complains of pain 10 minutes after a SC injection of morphine and asks for another injection. You:

   a. tell him you will give him another injection now
   b. tell him that the injection has not yet had a chance to work
   c. tell him he must wait another 2 hours
   d. tell him he must wait another 3 hours

36. A patient is ordered 10 mg oxycodone 'strictly 4-hourly'. When the patient's next dose is due it is noted that she has a sedation score of 2. You decide the best course of action is to:

   a. withhold the dose
   b. give 5 mg oxycodone only
   c. give naloxone
   d. give the oxycodone as ordered

37. An 80-year-old patient is given 15 mg oral oxycodone. One hour later she is noted to have a sedation score of 3. You are asked to give naloxone. An appropriate dose and route would be:

   a. 40–100 µg naloxone IM
   b. 40–100 µg naloxone IV
   c. 400 µg naloxone IV
   d. 100 mg naloxone IV

38. A continuous infusion of morphine is ordered at a rate of 2 mg/h. On average, the full effect of morphine given at that rate of infusion will be seen within:

   a. 15 minutes
   b. 1 hour
   c. 4 hours
   d. 15 hours

39. Transdermal fentanyl patches enable fentanyl to be absorbed through the skin. These patches:

   a. have an effect that may last 24 hours after the patch is removed
   b. allow blood concentrations of fentanyl to rise rapidly
   c. are useful in the routine management of acute pain
   d. have only small amounts of fentanyl left in the patch after removal

40. A patient using PCA with a bolus dose of 2 mg morphine (lockout 6 minutes) complains of repeatedly waking in severe pain at night. He is receiving, on average, 8 mg every hour (i.e. four 'successful' demands). You would:

   a. tell him to press the demand button more frequently, as he can get more doses from the machine each hour
   b. suspect he has an addiction to morphine
   c. tell him that an increase in the size of the bolus dose is not appropriate
   d. consider the use of a continuous (background) infusion

41. A patient using PCA with a bolus dose of 2 mg morphine (lockout 6 minutes) complains of severe pain. He is receiving, on average, 8 mg every hour (i.e. four 'successful' demands). He has a sedation score of 2. You would:

   a. tell him to press the demand button more frequently, as he can get more doses from the machine each hour
   b. reduce the size of the bolus dose
   c. increase the lockout interval
   d. consider the use of a continuous (background) infusion

42. A patient using PCA morphine complains of severe itching over his face and chest. A decision is made to change to PCA fentanyl. If the bolus dose of morphine is currently 1 mg, an appropriate bolus dose of fentanyl would be:

   a. 1 μg
   b. 5 μg
   c. 20 μg
   d. 50 μg

43. The following statements are true about IV patient-controlled analgesia EXCEPT:

   a. antireflux valves should be used unless a dedicated line is available for PCA
   b. antisiphon valves should always be used in the line between a patient and drug reservoir
   c. the dose cannot be altered in disposable PCA devices
   d. the record of the number of 'successful' versus 'unsuccessful' bolus dose deliveries is a useful guide to alterations in the size of the dose

44. The following statements are true about IV patient-controlled analgesia EXCEPT:

   a. changing the lockout interval has been shown to improve pain relief
   b. use of a 4-hourly dose limit will not necessarily prevent overdose of PCA opioid
   c. smaller bolus doses may be appropriate in older patients
   d. the routine use of a background infusion increases the risk of respiratory depression

45. A dose of epidural morphine that gives a similar degree of pain relief as 5 mg IM morphine is:

   a. 0.1 mg
   b. 0.5 mg
   c. 1 mg
   d. 5 mg

46. A dose of intrathecal morphine that gives a similar degree of pain relief as 5 mg IM morphine is:

   a. 0.1 mg
   b. 0.5 mg
   c. 1 mg
   d. 5 mg

47. Epidural opioids cause:

   a. less nausea and vomiting than epidural local anesthetics
   b. more itching than epidural local anesthetics
   c. more hypotension than epidural local anesthetics
   d. less sedation than epidural local anesthetics

48. Postdural puncture headache is typically:

   a. bifrontal or occipital
   b. usually worse when lying down than when sitting
   c. a result of leakage of blood into the epidural space
   d. more likely in older patients

49. The following statements about a patient with an epidural abscess are true EXCEPT:

   a. the patient will always require surgery
   b. the patient may have no neurological signs
   c. the patient may be afebrile
   d. the patient presents with increasing back pain

50. A patient with an epidural abscess accompanied by leg weakness will have the best chance of full recovery if diagnosis and treatment are carried out within:

   a. 8 hours of the onset of leg weakness
   b. 12 hours of the onset of leg weakness
   c. 18 hours of the onset of leg weakness
   d. 24 hours of the onset of leg weakness

51. A patient is receiving an epidural infusion of bupivacaine 0.1% and fentanyl 5 μg/mL at a rate of 10 mL/h for postoperative analgesia. His operation was 2 days ago. He tells you that he has some numbness in both legs. You would:

    a. tell him that it is likely to be due to the bupivacaine
    b. cease the infusion or reduce the rate of infusion
    c. consider the possibility of epidural hematoma or epidural abscess
    d. all of the above

52. A patient is receiving an epidural infusion of bupivacaine 0.1% and fentanyl 5 μg/mL at a rate of 7 mL/h for postoperative analgesia. His operation was 2 days ago. You note that his blood pressure is 80 mmHg systolic (it had been 130). You would:

    a. tell him that it is likely to be due to the bupivacaine
    b. administer naloxone
    c. consider the possibility of postoperative bleeding
    d. all of the above

53. A patient calls you from her home at 10 pm. She has increasing back pain and is having trouble voiding. She says that you gave her an epidural anesthetic for her hysterectomy 5 weeks ago. You would:

    a. tell her to come to your hospital first thing tomorrow morning
    b. tell her that she must come to the hospital for immediate assessment
    c. tell her to see her general practitioner
    d. tell her that back pain is a common problem after epidural anesthesia and that she should take two paracetamol (acetaminophen) tablets every 4 hours and call again in the morning

54. An increased risk of phantom pain is associated with all of the following EXCEPT:

    a. male gender
    b. severe preamputation pain
    c. chemotherapy
    d. severe postoperative stump pain

55. A patient is admitted following a motorbike accident. He has no movement in his right arm and an injury to his brachial plexus is suspected. Four days later he says that he has burning and shooting pains in his arm. He also says that the morphine he is getting is not helping the pain nearly as much as it was before. This type of pain is called:

    a. nociceptive pain
    b. neuropathic pain
    c. psychological pain
    d. phantom pain

56. Phantom pain:

   a. is more likely to occur days to weeks after limb amputation than within the first few days
   b. is more likely after a traumatic amputation
   c. is not prevented by the perioperative use of ketamine
   d. may respond to ketamine, gabapentin and calcitonin

57. Preventive analgesia:

   a. means than an analgesic drug or technique given before an intervention (e.g. surgical incision) results in less pain than with the technique drug given after the intervention
   b. means that the analgesic effect of a drug or technique exceeds the expected duration of effect
   c. is not seen with ketamine
   d. has not been seen with epidural analgesia

58. Strategies that may help to improve postoperative analgesia in opioid-tolerant patient include all of the following EXCEPT:

   a. the addition of non-opioid analgesics such as NSAIDs and paracetamol
   b. use of ketamine
   c. use of a benzodiazepine
   d. use of regional analgesic techniques

59. Patients in a substance abuse treatment program may be prescribed methadone, buprenorphine or naltrexone. All of the following statements about their treatment when presenting for surgery are true EXCEPT:

   a. methadone regimens should be continued where possible
   b. naltrexone regimens should be continued where possible
   c. buprenorphine regimens may be continued where possible
   d. they may require treatment for withdrawal from other drugs, such as benzodiazepines

60. In patients with mild renal impairment it is reasonable to use all of the following EXCEPT:

   a. fentanyl
   b. oxycodone
   c. pethidine (meperidine)
   d. buprenorphine

Answers

1. b	23. d	45. c
2. d	24. a	46. a
3. a	25. c	47. b
4. b	26. b	48. a
5. c	27. b	49. a
6. b	28. a	50. a
7. a	29. a	51. d
8. c	30. b	52. c
9. a	31. a	53. b
10. d	32. c	54. a
11. b	33. c	55. b
12. d	34. b	56. d
13. c	35. b	57. b
14. c	36. a	58. c
15. d	37. b	59. b
16. b	38. d	60. c
17. a	39. a	
18. c	40. d	
19. c	41. b	
20. c	42. c	
21. a	43. d	
22. d	44. a	

Index